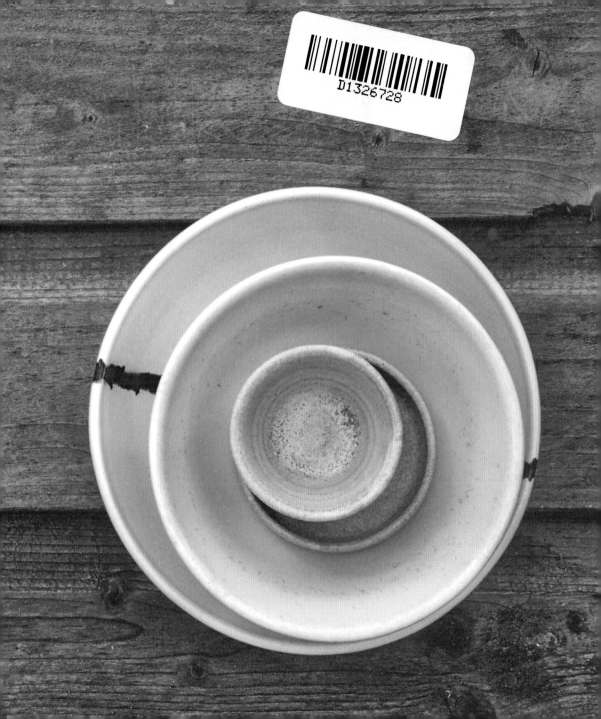

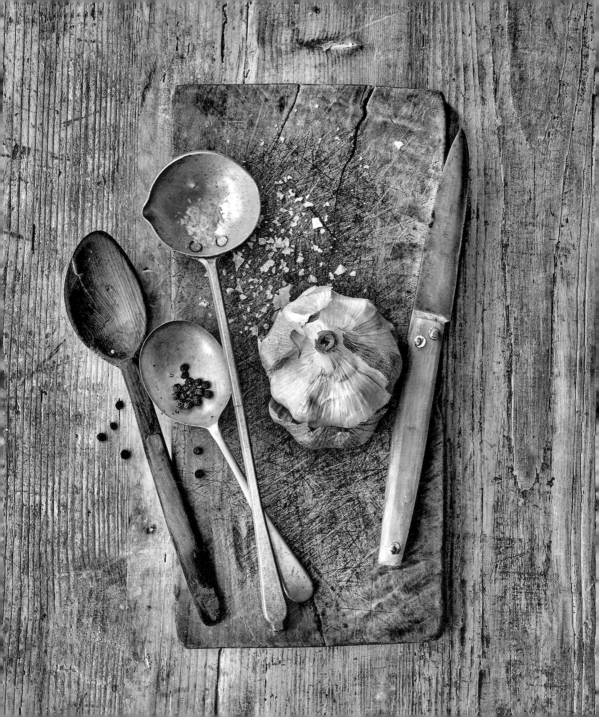

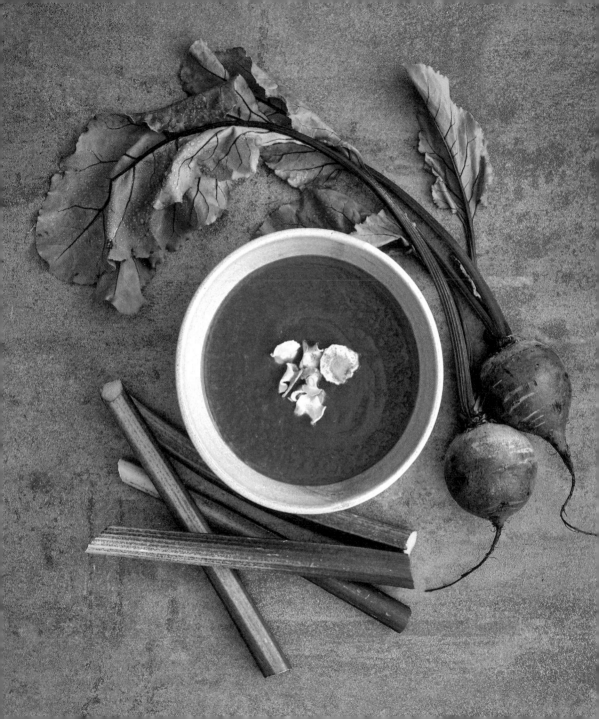

soupologie

PLANT-BASED, GLUTEN-FREE SOUPS TO HEAL, CLEANSE & ENERGISE

STEPHEN ARGENT

Vermilion
LONDON

10 9 8 7 6 5 4 3 2 1

Vermilion, an imprint of Ebury Publishing,
20 Vauxhall Bridge Road,
London SW1V 2SA

Vermilion is part of the Penguin Random House
group of companies whose addresses can be found
at global.penguinrandomhouse.com

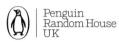

Penguin
Random House
UK

First published in the United Kingdom
by Vermilion in 2017

www.penguin.co.uk

A CIP catalogue record for this book is available from
the British Library

ISBN 9781785040955

Printed and bound in China by Toppan Leefung

Penguin Random House is committed to a sustainable future
for our business, our readers and our planet. This book is
made from Forest Stewardship Council ® certified paper

MIX
Paper from
responsible sources
FSC
www.fsc.org   FSC® C018179

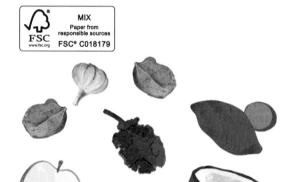

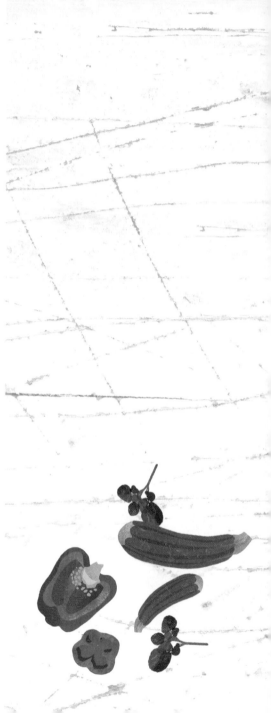

CONTENTS

INTRODUCTION

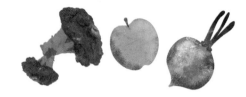

Welcome to the world of delicious, health-giving soups. I am the founder of Soupologie, the UK's leading plant-based, free-from, fresh soup company, and I am excited to share with you my passion for nutritious, homemade soups. Gone are the days when soup was something you had as a bit of comfort food, to keep you going until the 'real' food arrived. Now, through the use of some carefully chosen ingredients and a dash of imagination, the possibilities for nourishing and tasty soups are endless.

In this book, I shall be showing you how soups can become a staple in your diet, so you can benefit from their high nutrient value and their low energy density – this means that you get lots of key nutrients for relatively few calories. Soupologie soups are vegan, dairy-free and gluten-free, and packed with fresh vegetables to ensure that each soup has as much goodness as possible.

The one principle that I stick to is that, no matter what your diet regime or how motivated you are to eat well, you will always compromise your diet if the food you're eating isn't enjoyable and satisfying. So you'll find that all the recipes in this book are as tasty as they are good for you.

The first section of the book is about 'souping'. We're all guilty of some over-indulgences now and again, as well as grabbing snacks on the go and

wolfing down food that's convenient but not very good for us. So we devised the souping plans as a warming and highly replenishing way to give your digestive system a rest. The plans are not about deprivation or calorie counting, but nourishing your body with the nutrients it needs to rebuild and recharge. With the help of our dietitians we have put together a complete programme, which includes a regime to follow before following a souping plan as well as a gentle easing back to eating a wider variety of foods again. The one-, three- and five-day plans should provide you with all the nourishment you need to keep full and satiated with a sense of wellbeing.

The introductory section is followed by a variety of lovingly created recipes to give you an all-year-round collection of soups. They will enhance your wellbeing with their wide range of restorative nutrients, whose health benefits are clearly indicated by the small icons above each recipe.

We don't need to strive for perfection, we just need to help our bodies feel great by eating well. Here's to your Souper Powers!

Stephen

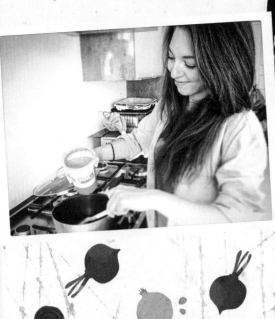

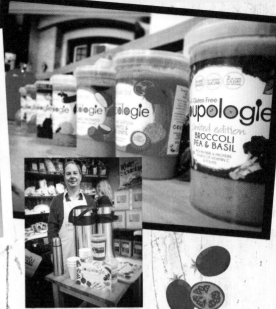

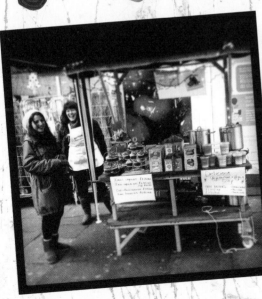

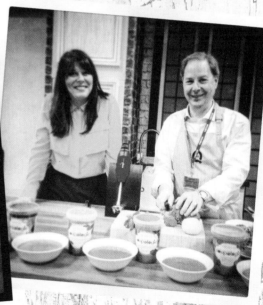

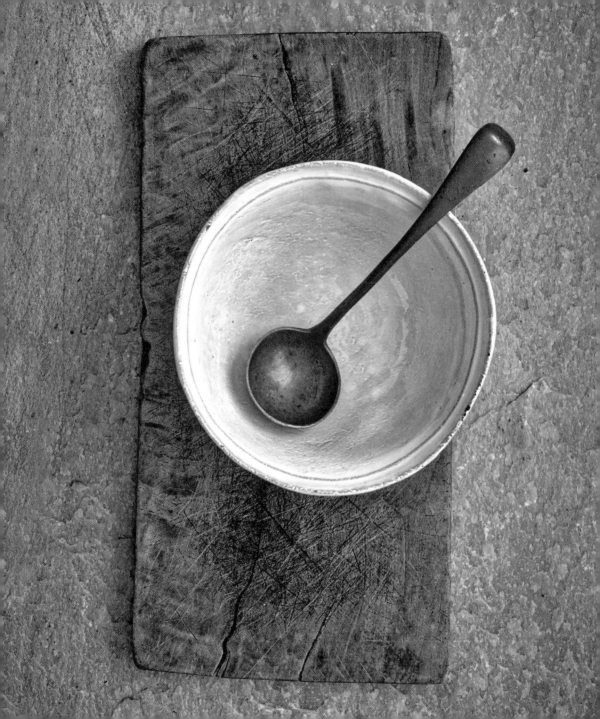

THE SOUPOLOGIE PLAN

Whether you're recovering from a period of excess, preparing for holiday sun, or feel that your body needs a nutrient boost, our souping plans step up to the plate (or bowl!). We all know veggies are good for us, yet most of us aren't getting what we need. So commit to one, three or five days of nourishing plant power with our souping plans to give your digestive system a break and keep your immune system strong.

THE SOUPOLOGIE STORY

I started making soups for my family many years ago when my four daughters were little and supermarket soups were more likely to taste of chemicals than vegetables. As the children grew up, they went through a phase of clamouring for junk food, but then started to become more interested in what they were eating, gradually developing ideas and tastes of their own. Meanwhile my wife Amanda and I became more interested in understanding the relationship between food, diet and healthy eating and our own wellbeing. I sought out better-quality ingredients, cut down on certain foods that seemed to be less healthy and read about the power of great nutrition. It didn't take long to realise that eating healthily and responsibly directly affects how you feel physically, and often emotionally too.

Soupologie started when I was encouraged by friends and family to take my homemade soups to a local Christmas Fair. Armed with a couple of large saucepans, one filled with Tomato and Red Lentil Soup (see page 84) and the other with Roasted Butternut and Red Pepper Soup (see page 100), I was overwhelmed by how quickly the soups sold, and the wonderful compliments I received about the flavours. What started out as an adventure to revolutionise the soup market with my Soupologie fresh soup brand, packing as much nutrition as possible into every pot, has led to many insights for me into food, sensible eating and superfood ingredients. I am thrilled to be able to share my knowledge and recipes with you here.

WHY SOUP?

Over the years, it's driven me crazy that soup has become the Cinderella of the food world: it has largely been ignored, pushed around and treated harshly. Commercial soups are often stuffed with artificial thickeners, sugar, milk, cream, cheap cuts of meat, maltodextrin, glucose syrup — and that's just the fresh soup! Sure, these soups will make you feel full because there's so much water content, but the nutritional value is next to nothing and the taste has to be pepped up with flavourings.

My philosophy is that soups should be naturally flavoursome and healthy, rich in nutrients and packed with superfood ingredients to provide food that is filling, delicious and good for you. In fact, I believe that soups should be good for everyone, from kids to grandparents and anyone in between. They should be crammed full of vegetables that include vital fibre, which makes you feel full, soothes your digestive system and keeps your blood sugar steady. Don't get me wrong,

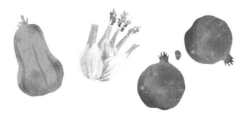

"I get lots of my inspiration from my four daughters, who are renowned for challenging me, especially in the early days of Soupologie, to make soups with unusual ingredients that were way outside of my comfort zone. I am eternally grateful to them for sometimes pushing my creativity to its limits. With the devil-may-care attitude of youth, they have taught me not to back away from a challenge, but instead rise to it with gusto! There are so many wonderful and exotic vegetables, fruits, herbs and spices out there that I would urge you all to have a go and test your tastebuds."

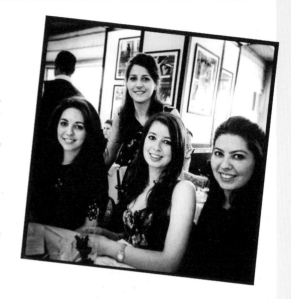

I am all for using up the veg knocking around at the back of your fridge, but with this book I want to show you how the clever use of some highly nourishing, sometimes novel ingredients can turn a bowl of soup into a nutritional powerhouse. You're standing over a hot stove making soup anyway, so why not turn it into the most potent, health-giving bowl of goodness possible?

PLANNING FOR HEALTH

Many people have found that they really benefit from doing short cleanses, over periods of one, three or five days, but this needs to be done in a healthy, structured way to make sure you feel well and pleasantly full, rather than deprived. So Team Soupologie have helped me to devise three unique souping plans that will allow you to pick and mix your favourite recipes, flavours and ingredients from a few simple tables, and actually enjoy your cleanse while instantly feeling its benefits. With the help of Sian Porter, our nutritionist, we have also added in healthy snacking options to keep you totally happy, energised and satiated all day.

If you plan your 'plan', so to speak, you'll find that souping is a really efficient way of managing a cleansing or detoxing period. Set aside half a day to do all the cooking and you'll be able to make enough soup to last you through your chosen daily programme, whether this is one, three or five days, with plenty left over for the freezer. This means that your half-day soup-cooking fest should carry you through several souping plans over the course of the following few months.

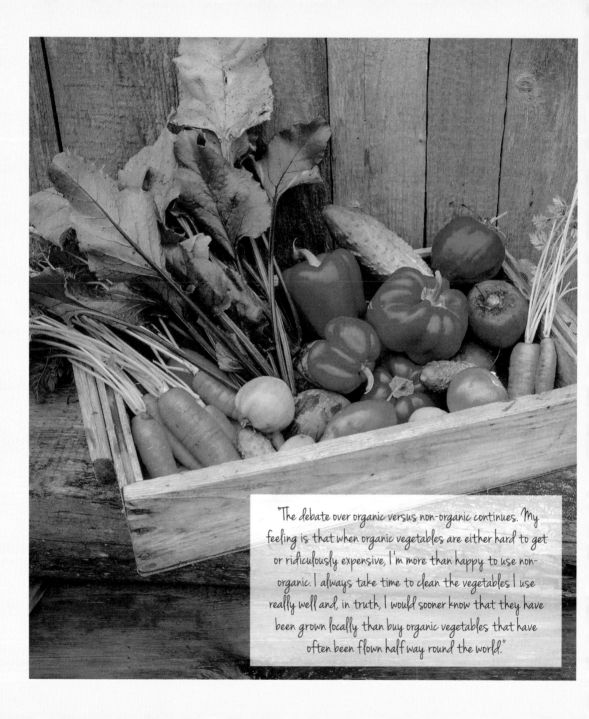

"The debate over organic versus non-organic continues. My feeling is that when organic vegetables are either hard to get or ridiculously expensive, I'm more than happy to use non-organic. I always take time to clean the vegetables I use really well and, in truth, I would sooner know that they have been grown locally than buy organic vegetables that have often been flown half way round the world."

THE SOUPING PLANS

At Soupologie, we are fans of plant power and the way that plant-based soups can help you feel and look good from the inside out. Gone are the days of starving yourself in an attempt to look better. We believe that you should take care of your body without having to make too many sacrifices or suffering discomfort along the way. This means nourishing, not punishing, your body and allowing the comforting and healthy benefits of fresh soups to bring you all the goodness you need.

Hearty, healthy soups have long been part of a balanced eating programme but this book will allow you to enjoy the benefits of soup as a dedicated, nutritionally designed programme from the comfort of your own home. We have done all the hard work for you, by creating soups that bring you the very best blend of seasonal, plant-based ingredients, harnessing all their goodness without compromising on taste.

Whether you are keen to give your digestive system a rest, or simply enjoy a menu of warming soups, our one-, three- and five-day souping plans bring you a balance of protein, fibre and phytonutrients (natural plant chemicals with antioxidant and anti-inflammatory properties that may also improve intercellular communications and repair DNA damage). The US Department of Agriculture says that eating phytonutrient-rich foods seems to be an 'effective strategy'

for lowering the risk of cancer and heart disease, which is also why the World Health Organization (WHO) recommend that we eat more than 400 g (14 oz) per day of fresh fruit and vegetables. The powerful mix of protein, fibre and phytonutrients begins to deliver benefits immediately, as it gently helps the body to do its job of eliminating waste and toxins whilst maintaining energy levels and keeping blood sugar steady.

So much of our diet today consists of processed foods lacking an identified origin and often containing high levels of sugar, poor-quality ingredients, chemical additives and preservatives. This accumulation of poor nutrition has long been suspected to contribute to fatigue, weight gain, gastrointestinal distress and other ill-effects that impact upon our good health and, consequently, our longevity.

A plant-based diet has been scientifically shown to have impressive potential health benefits. These are not necessarily reduced during the cooking process – some phytonutrients in vegetables, such as carotenoids in carrots and spinach, actually need cooking to maximise their nutritional value. The digestibility of food, especially of plant foods, is also aided by cooking or pureeing the food. Good soup, it seems, is the perfect health food.

CHOOSING YOUR PLAN

Our souping plans have been designed around the recipes that form the second section of this book. Together with the pre- and post- cleanse advice, they form the basis of a nutritionally balanced cleansing program. You can follow the plans as laid out here, or you can build your own using the assortment of soups across the tables, according to your personal taste and preferences.

We have named the one-day plan the 'Rest-day Plan', as this has been created for those days when you want to give your system just that: a day of rest. We find the Rest-day Plan is the perfect antidote to an over-indulgent weekend and a great way to re-set your eating habits. This plan draws on powerful science showing how short periods of fasting, if properly controlled, can achieve a number of health benefits.

The three-day and five-day plans are comprehensive ways to help your body help itself, by flooding it with active, living macro- and micro-nutrients. Soups are essentially a blend of foods already broken down, which may help the body to focus on healing itself and making bigger strides in building strength. These plans allow you to enjoy all the healthy benefits of whole vegetables including their naturally occurring fibrous skins, seeds and flesh. This is one of the ways in which the soups outclass juice cleanses, which are popular at the moment. Juicing removes the truly nutritious fibrous skin and pulp that we need to help stay healthy, and juice cleanses based on sweet fruits can lead to a spike in blood sugar levels without the buffering qualities of fibre and pulp. In contrast to juice, the dietary fibre in soup fills you up and slows digestion, so that the natural sugars from the carbohydrates are absorbed more slowly into the bloodstream. The fibre in a bowl of soup naturally reduces the Glycaemic Index (GI) and glycaemic load of a meal. Lower GI diets are associated with decreased risk of certain diseases and optimising health, and they may help to control appetite.

Our fibre-filled soups can also aid weight loss in the safe, sound manner that the medical community recommends. Each recipe is free from gluten, dairy, processed soy and refined sugar.

Some of the possible benefits are listed below:
- Weight loss and reduction of bloating
- Better bowel function
- More energy and less fatigue
- Improved mood
- Decreased gastrointestinal problems
- Better digestion
- Increased nutrients
- Increased immune system support
- Healthy skin and hair.

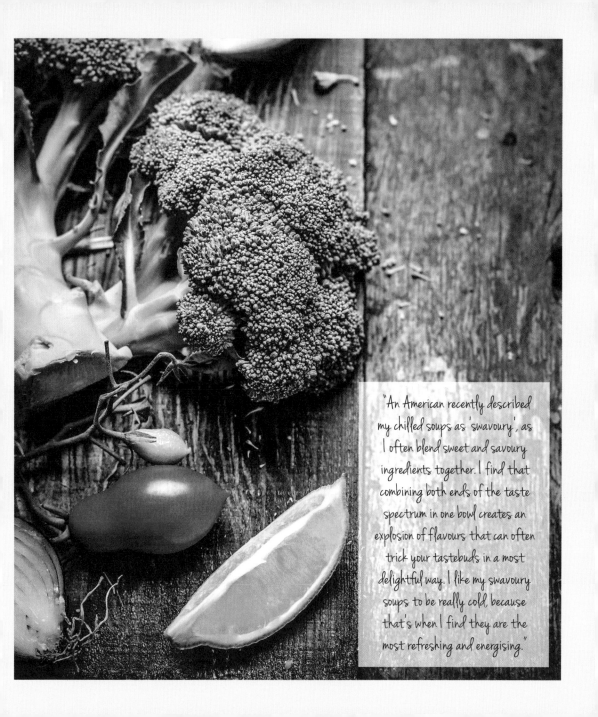

"An American recently described my chilled soups as 'swavoury', as I often blend sweet and savoury ingredients together. I find that combining both ends of the taste spectrum in one bowl creates an explosion of flavours that can often trick your tastebuds in a most delightful way. I like my swavoury soups to be really cold, because that's when I find they are the most refreshing and energising."

"Be wary of products that use the word 'skinny'. It's not about skinny, it's about eating for health and wellbeing, about resting your digestive system and not overloading it with processed foods. Always look for foods that are made with healthy ingredients, without added sugars, lots of salt or artificial thickeners, and that way you don't need to calorie-count. If you're eating healthily and nourishing your body, your weight will take care of itself."

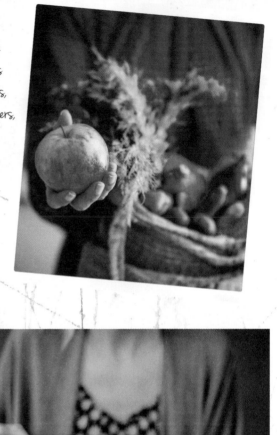

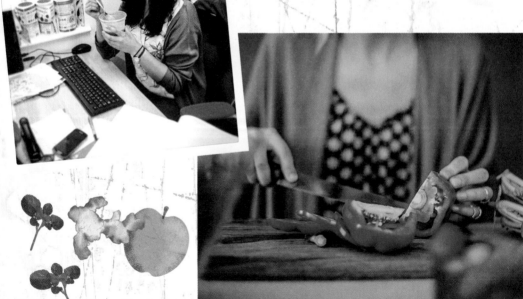

BEFORE YOU START

It is important to note that the souping plans on the following pages may help improve your health and wellbeing but we do not claim to 'treat' or 'cure' any disease. If you have any concerns regarding undertaking a soup cleanse, please consult your doctor or another medical or complementary health practitioner before you start. None of the information supplied in this book is intended as a substitute for the advice of a doctor or healthcare professional.

While every care has been taken to ensure the suitability of the programme for the majority of people's needs, there are some exceptions. Our soup cleanses are naturally low in calories, so should not be undertaken by women who are breast-feeding or pregnant, or the elderly. If you are on medication or have an existing or chronic medical condition such as Type 1 diabetes, please check with your doctor first. Similarly, if you are taking supplements or other natural remedies, please consult with your complementary health practitioner to check that there are no contra-indications in following the souping plan. The soup cleanses may not be suitable for people with a nut allergy or other allergy that can result in anaphylactic shock.

Our cleansing plans form a specialist programme that should be treated as such. They are not intended for permanent or long-term use.

THE TRANSITION PHASE

It is important that you prepare well for your soup cleanse, so that you can truly reap all the benefits. Whether you intend to follow the one-, three- or five-day plan, the way you will be eating is likely to be very different from what your body is used to. For this reason we do not advise diving in at the deep end straight away. Begin, instead, by giving your body a gentle introduction to a new way of eating by allowing yourself a short 'transition phase'. This involves phasing out certain types of foods and undertaking a few lifestyle changes, as described over the following pages.

The transition stage can be used to make the cleanse that follows a more enjoyable and effective experience. Follow the guidelines on pages 18 and 19 for as many days as possible before starting your chosen plan; as an absolute minimum, follow them on the day before your plan starts. Preparation is key, so make it a priority to ensure that you are giving your body the best possible start on this journey to better health.

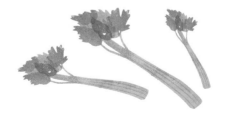

INCREASE YOUR SLEEP

Sleep is essential for renewal and rejuvenation of your body's cells. As a rule, you should aim to achieve eight to nine hours of shut-eye every night to support your immune system and nourish your cognitive health.

WHAT TO EAT BEFORE YOUR CLEANSE

During the transition phase, allow your body to start adjusting to a healthier way of eating by doing as many of the following as you can:

• Choose fresh produce wherever possible.
• Eat a high proportion of fruit and vegetables.
• Aim to eat at least eight different types of fruit or vegetables per day.
• Try to vary your diet as much as possible, within the confines of this transitional stage.
• Eat lots of highly nutritious leafy green vegetables.
• Eat at least every four hours to balance blood-sugar levels.
• Include a small amount of protein with every meal.

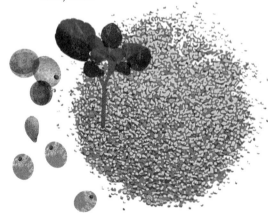

• Don't go hungry: if you feel starving you are likely to make inappropriate food choices.
• Eat only wholefoods (foods that are natural and unprocessed).
• Minimise the eating of ready prepared and refined foods, especially products made with white flour and white rice; replace these with wholemeal flour and wild or brown rice.
• Reduce your intake of animal produce and increase your intake of vegetable proteins such as pulses.
• Eat slowly and chew your food thoroughly.
• Say goodbye to sugar. Five days before starting on any of the plans, cut out the obvious sources of sugar, such as ready meals, chocolate, sweets, biscuits and the biggie: alcohol. Whatever your tipple of choice, alcohol will dehydrate you and it can increase the risk of medical conditions such as certain forms of cancer, strokes and raised blood pressure.
• Think 'plain and simple'. Five days before starting our plan, keep your diet simple with easy-to-prepare-from-scratch foods. Think porridge with berries and seeds for breakfast, baked sweet potato (with oily fish if you aren't vegan) and salad for lunch, and bean soup with steamed veggies for dinner.
• Try to incorporate at least one mixed green side salad per day and three servings of fresh fruit.

We find that all of these are made easier by preparing a shopping list before shopping, so it's less easy to be distracted by treats.

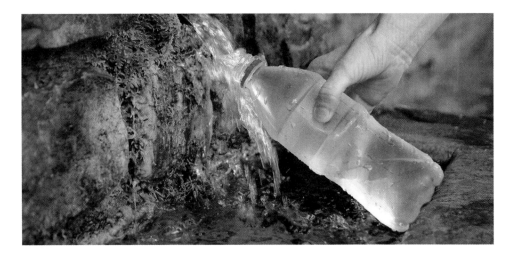

Listed below are some ideas for appropriate meals during the transition stage.

BREAKFAST

- Berries with unsweetened Greek yoghurt and a small handful of mixed nuts or seeds.
- Oat porridge with almond milk and grated apple.
- Two boiled eggs on gluten-free bread or oatcakes (this option is good if you're looking for a high-protein breakfast).

LUNCH/DINNER

- Your choice of any of our soup recipes plus a green side salad with avocado.
- Poached or grilled fish with plenty of steamed vegetables of your choice.
- Stir-fried or steamed vegetables with wild rice.
- Baked sweet potato with goat's cheese plus a green side salad.

SNACKS

The following snacks are good to eat during the transition phase and during any of the plans:

- Rice cakes or oatcakes with cashew or almond nut butter, eaten with half a banana.
- Half an avocado spread on a slice of rye bread.
- An apple and a handful of unsalted seeds or nuts.
- Raw carrots, celery, cucumber, peppers, cherry tomatoes, cauliflower florets.
- A small bowl of natural bio/live yoghurt.
- Plain popcorn (no added salt or sugar).

DRINKS

Keep your body hydrated with water; around 2 litres (3½ pints) per day should be about right. This will make you feel more awake, increase your concentration and help reduce headaches. Cut caffeine gradually by half a cup per day, to avoid withdrawal headaches.

GETTING MORE FROM YOUR PLAN

There are several ways in which you can increase the effectiveness of the Soupologie plans and help your body along to better health and fitness fast but safely. Gentle exercise and physical stimulation can help to boost circulation, reawaken a sluggish digestive system, eliminate toxins and help the body relax at a deeper level.

The following ideas may be useful while you are following a three- or five-day Soupologie plan:

• Wake your body: kick-start your digestive system by drinking a cup or glass of warm water with lemon first thing.

• Body brush: dry-brush before your bath or shower, starting from the soles of your feet and moving upwards, as this boosts the circulation.

• Sip water regularly: continue to drink 2 litres (3½ pints) of water and add in some nurturing, caffeine-free herbal teas, such as nettle, dandelion, fennel or chamomile. Sip these slowly. Make a batch of fresh vegan broth (recipe on page 43) to sip throughout the day. This recipe yields a substantial, savoury stock-like broth that is perfect for filling those mid-morning and late-afternoon hunger-pang moments.

• Take an Epsom salt bath: have a hot bath or foot soak with Epsom salts in the evening to treat your skin and help your body relax.

• Avoid strenuous exercise but introduce gentle movement: consider introducing your body to some gentle yoga or stretching, or go for a swim or a walk.

• Use the power of steam: you could make use of your local gym's sauna or steam room (not for too long) to help eliminate toxins via the skin.

• Treat yourself: book a relaxing or lymphatic-drainage massage. Alternatively, have a facial or try some relaxing acupuncture.

POST-SOUPING

Just as you eased yourself into the Soupologie plan with a transitional phase, it's a good idea to follow your plan by easing yourself gently back to eating a wider range of foods. The following post-souping tips will also help maximise your results:

• Take it slowly: ease yourself back into three meals a day gradually, keeping the good stuff in your diet as much as possible. Leafy salads, soups and roasted veggies are all excellent choices.

• Rainbow-up your diet: eat something brightly coloured and green at every meal (think beetroot, carrots, peppers, aubergines, tomatoes, kale, spinach, broccoli, watercress) as these veggies can really help to keep your body happy.

- Eat fermented foods: gut-friendly fermented foods like live yoghurt, sauerkraut and kimchi increase levels of healthy bacteria, which may help to keep bloating at bay.

- Get sweaty! Exercise is just what the body needs following an intense healthy-eating regime. A good sweat session helps to remove toxins from the body, so combine high-intensity workouts like running or cycling (for boosting metabolism) with low-key yoga (for stretching and stamina) to give yourself perfectly balanced exercise.

- Stay off sugar: if you find it difficult to control your sweet tooth once you have finished the plan, try swapping to fruit and replacing chemical sweeteners and refined sugar with Stevia. This naturally sweet plant extract won't spike insulin levels or create any of the roller-coaster energy crashes that come with regular sugar.

- Fast occasionally: fasting, done sensibly and in moderation, gives your body a much-needed time-out to heal itself. Recent clinical trials have shown that fast days can have an important impact on your wellbeing. A 2014 research paper by Mattson, Allison, et al. on the frequency and daily timing of meals found that the introduction of intermittent energy-restriction periods – of as little as 16 hours – can improve health indicators and counteract disease processes. This seems to be due to a metabolic shift and the stimulation of certain stress responses that work to prevent and repair cellular damage.

If you're ready to get started, choose one of our unique plans outlined on the following pages. Eating this way will provide you with an easy way to cut out less-healthy foods and flood your body with easily digestible and nutritious ingredients.

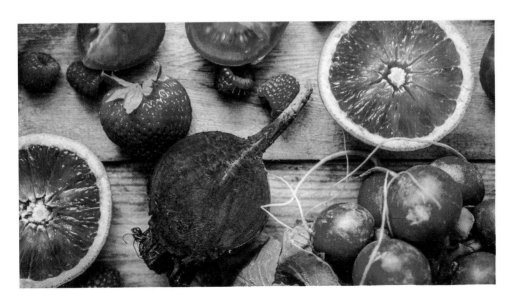

THE REST-DAY PLAN

We have created the 24-hour 'Rest-day' plan to provide you with a collection of light, fresh-tasting soups that you can eat over the course of just one day for a short but effective cleanse. This plan ensures that you obtain just the right balance of nutrients and avoid bloating. The soups have also been created to help you feel full and satisfied throughout the day, and ultimately leave you feeling 'rested', making the plan a prerequisite for the perfect day off.

Please note that our tables use the reference term 'NRV' (Nutrient Reference Value), which has replaced (but is equal to) the old-style 'RDA' (Recommended Daily Allowance).

	SOUP	POTENTIAL HEALTH BENEFITS	NUTRITIONAL INFORMATION (per 300 g/10½ oz serving)
MORNING	Beetroot and Orange (page 150)	Boosts immunity; relieves fatigue; stabilises blood sugar. Packed with folate for a healthy immune system and to help reduce tiredness and fatigue. Manganese content helps blood-sugar levels.	Energy: 201 kcal. Folate: 98% NRV, Manganese: 47% NRV. Protein: 1 g. Fibre: 3.9 g.
SNACK	Cucumber and Apple (page 56)	Quercetin in apples has been linked to anti-ageing; it is also said to have an anti-inflammatory action.	Energy: 186 kcal. Fibre: 3.3 g.
LUNCH	Broccoli Soup with Almond Pesto (page 134	Detoxifying, protein-rich and a good source of fibre. Broccoli contains phytochemicals that help to stimulate the body's detox systems.	Energy: 225 kcal. Vitamin C: 107% NRV, Folate: 45% NRV, Potassium: 20% NRV. Protein: 5.7 g. Fibre: 3.6 g.
SNACK	Tomato and Fennel Gazpacho (page 86)	Supports nervous system. High in lycopene, which has been linked to reduced risk of cancer, heart disease and age-related eye disorders.	Energy: 99 kcal. Potassium: 30% NRV, Vitamin C: 28% NRV. Fibre: 3.3 g. Protein: 2.4 g
DINNER	Golden Leek and Potato (page 122)	Aids digestion. Helps good bacteria to flourish in the gut. Boosts Vitamin B6, which helps regulate hormonal activity in the body.	Energy: 105 kcal. Vitamin B6: 36% NRV, Thiamin: 24% NRV. Fibre: 2.4 g. Protein: 2.4 g.

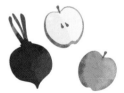

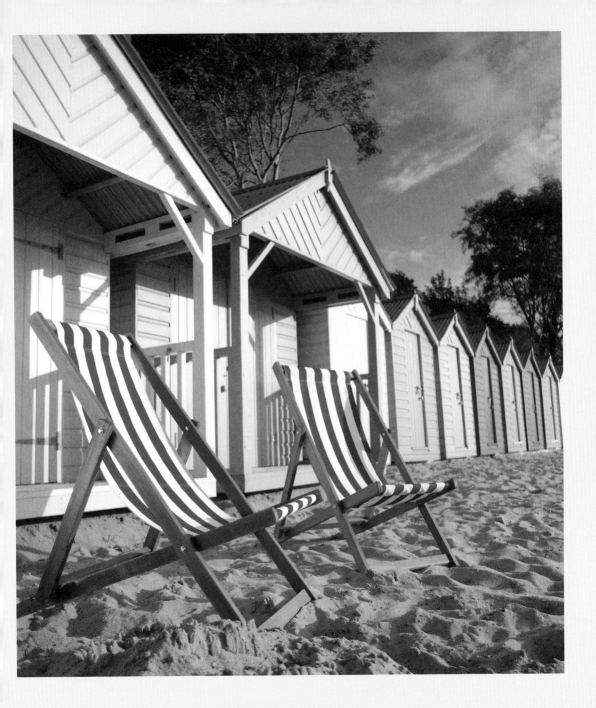

THE THREE-DAY PLAN

The soups in this plan have been carefully considered and selected for their various health-giving properties to ensure you are receiving the optimum nutrition for the time of day. We have personally tried and tested the soup-cleanse plans and have found that they are filling, enjoyable and leave you feeling energised and alert.

For ease of use, we have presented the plans in easy-to-follow tables that highlight the morning, lunch and dinner soup suggestions, while also providing you with a clear daily overview of the total number of calories, nutrients and fibre.

While following this plan, remember to:
- Eat 3–6 servings of soup per day.
- Drink a minimum of 2 litres (3½ pints) of water each day as well.
- Start each day with a large glass of warm water with a squeeze of lemon to hydrate and wake.
- Refer to the snacks given on page 19 if you feel the need for additional food during the day.

	SOUP	POTENTIAL HEALTH BENEFITS	NUTRITIONAL INFORMATION (per 300 g/10½ oz serving)
DAY 1			
MORNING	Mango, Melon and Coconut Soup (page 118)	Supports skin health; high in antioxidants. Fibre-rich mango provides a burst of betacarotene (converted in the body to Vitamin A) and Vitamin C. Cantaloupe is hydrating and boosts Vitamin A via betacarotene.	Energy: 135 kcal. Vitamin A: 71% NRV, Vitamin C: 95% NRV, Potassium: 26% NRV. Fibre: 3g.
LUNCH	Roasted Butternut and Red Pepper (page 100)	High in antioxidants; boosts metabolism; supports nervous system; maintains cardiovascular health. Contains Vitamin C, a powerful antioxidant. Rich in vitamins A (betacarotene) and E, as well as Vitamin B6 and folate, which help to support your metabolism and cardiovascular health, plus potassium for your nervous system.	Energy: 123 kcal. Vitamin A: 88% NRV, Vitamin C: 66% NRV, Vitamin E: 27% NRV, Folate: 18% NRV, Vitamin B6: 21% NRV. Fibre: 2.7 g.
DINNER	Mulligatawny (page 70)	Relaxing; aids sleep. Fibre- and protein-rich vegetable source of tryptophan, a sleep-aiding nutrient.	Energy: 261 kcal. Vitamin A: 42% NRV, Vitamin E: 29% NRV. Fibre: 4.5 g. Protein: 5.4 g.

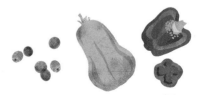

DAY 2

MORNING — Hearty Pea and Lentil (page 144)

Energy boosting; improves energy levels and gut health. High in protein and fibre with a boost of iron to power you up for the day ahead and copper to help you use it.

Energy: 201 kcal. Thiamin: 29% NRV, Vitamin C: 28% NRV, Vitamin B6: 24% NRV, Folate: 20% NRV, Potassium: 21% NRV, Iron: 25% NRV, Copper: 24%. Fibre: 3.6 g. Protein: 11.1 g.

LUNCH — Cauliflower and Mustard Seed (page 48)

High in antioxidants; detoxifying; improves energy levels. Cauliflower is low in sugars, fat and calories, yet high in Vitamin C, B6 and folate, in addition to containing Thiamin, Vitamin E, potassium, manganese and fibre. Like broccoli, cauliflower contains phytochemicals that help to stimulate the body's detox systems. The mustard seed adds protein and essential fats.

Energy: 132 kcal. Vitamin E 16% NRV, Vitamin C: 49% NRV, Thiamin: 19% NRV, Vitamin B6: 24% NRV, Folate: 32% NRV, Potassium: 21% NRV, Manganese: 16% NRV. Fibre: 3.3 g. Protein: 4.5 g.

DINNER — Minestrone (page 78)

Supports skin health; high in antioxidants; supports nervous system; improves energy levels. Being full of so many different vegetables, this soup has high amounts of vitamins A and E, as well as being a source of potassium and folate. The beans boost the fibre and protein content and the protective lycopene in the tomatoes is more easily absorbed when cooked.

Energy: 138 kcal. Vitamin A: 31% NRV, Vitamin E: 19% NRV, Vitamin C: 24% NRV, Potassium: 18% NRV, Folate: 32% NRV. Fibre: 3.9 g. Protein: 4.2 g.

DAY 3

MORNING — Carrot, Orange and Ginger (page 110)

Supports skin health; ginger aids digestion. Source of betacarotene (Vitamin A) which is more readily available from carrots when they have been cooked.

Energy: 129 kcal. Vitamin A: 126% NRV. Fibre: 3.3 g.

LUNCH — Courgette and Watercress Pesto (page 138)

Immune-boosting; supports nervous system. This light soup is packed with greens that care for your immune system with their Vitamin C content as well as potassium and B vitamins (thiamin, B6 and folate).

Energy: 138 kcal. Vitamin C: 31% NRV, Thiamin: 20% NRV, Vitamin B6: 23% NRV, Folate: 28% NRV, Potassium: 22%. Fibre: 2.4 g. Protein: 3.6 g.

DINNER — Tomato and Red Lentil (page 84)

High in antioxidants; low GI; maintains energy levels and supports skin health. Iron- and protein-rich, low-GI lentils keep blood levels steady. Contains immune-caring Vitamin C and skin-supportive vitamins A and E, in addition to B vitamins, keeping your energy levels and metabolism on track. High in potassium for bone and muscle health.

Energy: 162 kcal. Vitamin A: 26% NRV, Vitamin E: 23% NRV, Vitamin C: 15% NRV, Thiamin: 16% NRV, Vitamin B6: 19% NRV, Folate: 15% NRV, Potassium: 22% NRV. Fibre: 3 g. Protein: 5.7 g.

THE FIVE-DAY PLAN

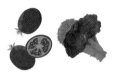

Make sure you read 'Before You Start' (on pages 17–19) before begining this programme. This will help ease you into the plan and feel its benefits from day one. Feel free to swap around soup flavours, as long as you consume at least the same number of calories and volume of liquid per day.

	SOUP	POTENTIAL HEALTH BENEFITS	NUTRITIONAL INFORMATION (per 300 g/10½ oz serving)
DAY 1			
MORNING	Raw Strawberry and Tarragon (page 90)	Aids digestion, high in antioxidants. Tarragon has traditionally been used to aid digestion. Source of Vitamin C as well as potassium and manganese. Strawberry seeds (on the outside of the fruit) are a good source of fibre.	Energy: 213 kcal. Vitamin C: 191% NRV, Folate: 21% NRV, Potassium: 19% NRV, Manganese: 28% NRV. Fibre: 6 g.
LUNCH	Potato and Summer Leaves (page 54)	High in antioxidants; aids digestion. Contains 20 g of carbohydrate per serving; includes vitamins C and B.	Energy: 159 kcal. Vitamin B6: 33% NRV, Thiamin: 22% NRV. Fibre: 2.4 g.
DINNER	Broccoli Soup with Almond Pesto (page 134)	Detoxifying; aids digestion; high in antioxidants. Supports healthy skin, hair and nails. This protein-rich soup will help keep you feeling full. Source of fibre. Broccoli contains phytochemicals that help stimulate the body's detox systems.	Energy: 225 kcal. Vitamin C: 107% NRV, Folate: 45% NRV. Fibre: 3.6g. Protein: 5.7 g.
DAY 2			
MORNING	Cucumber and Apple (page 56)	Anti-ageing; aids digestion. Quercetin in apples has been linked to anti-ageing and chloride to normal digestion.	Energy: 186 kcal. Chloride: 19% NRV. Fibre: 3.3 g.
LUNCH	Mushroom Soup (page 72)	Mushrooms are a source of protein and B vitamins that help in releasing energy from the food you eat. Copper helps look after skin and hair. You can make this soup with activated vitamin-D-rich mushrooms or leave them in the sun for that to do the job.	Energy: 126 kcal. Riboflavin (B2): 22% NRV, Niacin (B3): 21% NRV, Vitamin B6: 16% NRV, Folate: 24% NRV, Pantothenic acid: 33% NRV, Potassium: 18% NRV, Copper: 73% NRV. Fibre: 1.8 g. Protein: 4.8 g.
DINNER	London Particular (page 66)	High in fibre and protein, this soup will also provide a boost of iron for energy. Its thick, comforting depths contain lots of vitamins A and E too, which are great for supporting skin health.	Energy: 182 kcal. Vitamin A: 15% NRV, Vitamin E: 15% NRV, Vitamin B1: 27% NRV, Potassium: 18% NRV, Iron: 15% NRV, Manganese: 25% NRV,. Protein: 8.2 g. Fibre: 7.1 g.

DAY 3

MORNING	Tomato and Fennel Gazpacho (page 86)	Aids digestion; high in antioxidants; high in the protective carotenoid lycopene.	Energy: 99 kcal. Potassium: 30% NRV, Vitamin C: 28% NRV. Fibre: 3.3 g. Protein: 2.4 g.
LUNCH	Jerusalem Artichoke (page 46)	Aids digestion; supports gut health; relieves fatigue. This soup helps look after your digestive system by promoting beneficial gut bacteria and provides iron to keep blood healthy and reduce tiredness and fatigue.	Energy: 153 kcal. Vitamin A: 30% NRV, Vitamin E: 15% NRV, Thiamin: 22% NRV, Potassium: 22% NRV, Iron: 22% NRV. Fibre: 2.7 g. Protein: 2.7 g.
DINNER	Celeriac and Walnut (page 50)	Supports blood and bone health; high in antioxidants; contributes to brain health. This soup is a good source of Vitamin C, thiamin, Vitamin B6, folate, potassium and fibre.	Energy: 114 kcal. Vitamin C: 19% NRV, Thiamin: 20% NRV, Vitamin B6: 17% NRV, Folate: 24% NRV, Potassium: 23% NRV. Fibre: 2.4 g.

DAY 4

MORNING	Apricot Soup (page 116)	Aids digestion; good source of potassium, key player in keeping your brain, muscles and heart at the top of their game.	Energy: 126 kcal. Potassium: 56% NRV, Iron: 17% NRV, Copper: 24% NRV. Fibre: 5.4 g.
LUNCH	Parsnip and Apple (page 52)	Helps to protect cardiovascular health; high in antioxidants and fibre; anti-inflammatory. This soup is especially high in folate, a hard-working vitamin that protects cardiovascular health and contributes to a healthy immune system.	Energy: 141 kcal. Vitamin E: 20% NRV, Vitamin C: 22% NRV, Thiamin: 23% NRV, Folate: 40% NRV.
DINNER	Curried Parsnip and Sweet Potato (page 112)	High in fibre and antioxidants. Aids relaxation. The antioxidant vitamins C and E maximise the effect of the betacarotene and help with iron absorption.	Energy: 204 kcal. Vitamin E: 16% NRV, Vitamin C: 20% NRV, Thiamin: 20% NRV, Folate: 30% NRV, Potassium: 22% NRV, Iron 20% NRV, Manganese: 29% NRV. Fibre: 5.4 g. Protein: 3.3 g.

DAY 5

MORNING	Peach and Coconut Soup (page 126)	High in antioxidants; supports skin health. Contributes 93% of your NRV of Vitamin C and 15% of your recommended fibre intake for the day.	Energy: 162 kcal. Vitamin C: 93% NRV, Potassium: 18% NRV, Manganese: 21% NRV. Fibre: 4.5 g. Protein: 3 g.
LUNCH	Golden Leek and Potato (page 122)	Supports gut health and hormonal activity. Helps good bacteria to flourish in the gut. Boosts Vitamin B6, which helps regulate hormonal activity in the body.	Energy: 105 kcal. Vitamin B6: 36% NRV, Vitamin A: 36% NRV, Thiamin: 24% NRV. Fibre: 2.4 g. Protein: 2.4 g.
DINNER	Butterbean and Carrot (page 96)	Supports hair, skin and nails; boosts energy; aids digestion; high in antioxidants. High in protein, fibre and the ACE vitamins. Butterbeans are also a great source of protein and fibre.	Energy: 168 kcal. Vitamin A: 107% NRV, Vitamin E: 17% NRV, Vitamin C: 15% NRV, Folate: 23% NRV, Potassium: 24% NRV. Fibre: 5.7 g. Protein: 4.2 g.

FREQUENTLY ASKED QUESTIONS

Are the souping plans suitable for everyone?
The plans should be suitable for most healthy people but are not advised for children, pregnant and breast-feeding women, the elderly and those with an existing medical condition, or those with extremely physical occupations. This is because the soups are very low in calories. If in doubt, consult your doctor so that you can enjoy the plans with confidence.

Do I have to stick rigidly to a plan?
No! The soups can be eaten as an individual meal or snack, or as one day's worth of fresh, nutrient-rich meals, or as part of a Soupologie plan. Choose how you would like to eat the soups based on your tastes, needs and lifestyle, knowing that even one bowl of soup will provide you with high-quality nutrition and two servings of vegetables.

What side effects could there be?
Any changes in your usual lifestyle or food and drink choices can trigger changes in your body rhythms, resulting in mild symptoms, particularly if you are avoiding your usual caffeinated drinks. Headaches, changes in digestion and other symptoms could occur during the plans but these should settle and fade away. These are balanced nutritional plans that have been formulated to keep your metabolism and blood sugar steady. You are caring for yourself by consuming fibre-rich, whole fruits and vegetables with some wholegrains and

beans, not starving yourself. If you are worried about whether the plans may affect you adversely for any reason, particularly existing medical conditions, seek medical advice before starting.

Can I 'pick and mix' the recipes within each plan?
Of course. Just stick to the same portion size and don't skip any soup meals or snacks. If you would rather have a meal than soup in the evening, replace it with some lean protein or beans, wholegrains and lots of vegetables, gently cooked.

Must I eat the suggested amount of soup each day?
Yes, as the plans have been devised to give you the nutrition and energy you need. Skipping a meal or snack would reduce these. However, if you would rather have a meal in the evening, choose some lean protein or beans served with wholegrains and plenty of lightly cooked vegetables.

Can I add ingredients to the soups?
The plans are carefully designed to give you all the nourishment you need, but on pages 38–39 you'll find some ideas for 'souper toppers' that will add interesting texture and increase the nutritional value of the soups.

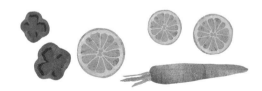

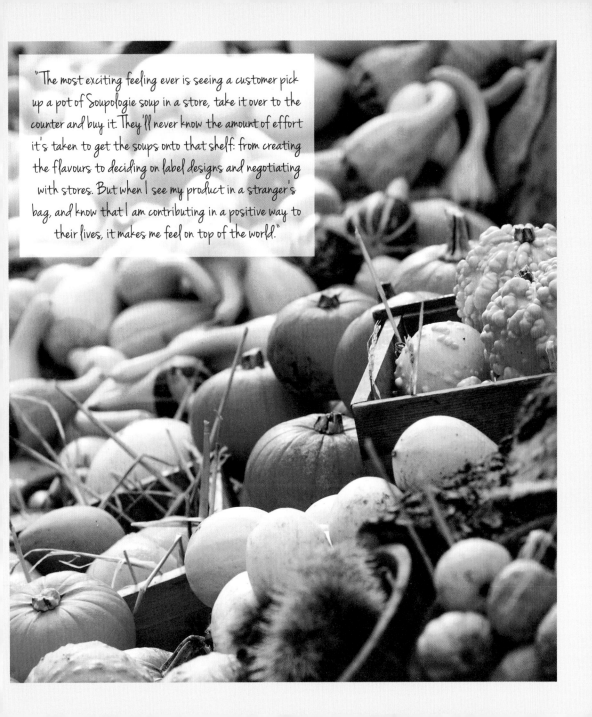

"The most exciting feeling ever is seeing a customer pick up a pot of Soupologie soup in a store, take it over to the counter and buy it. They'll never know the amount of effort it's taken to get the soups onto that shelf: from creating the flavours to deciding on label designs and negotiating with stores. But when I see my product in a stranger's bag, and know that I am contributing in a positive way to their lives, it makes me feel on top of the world."

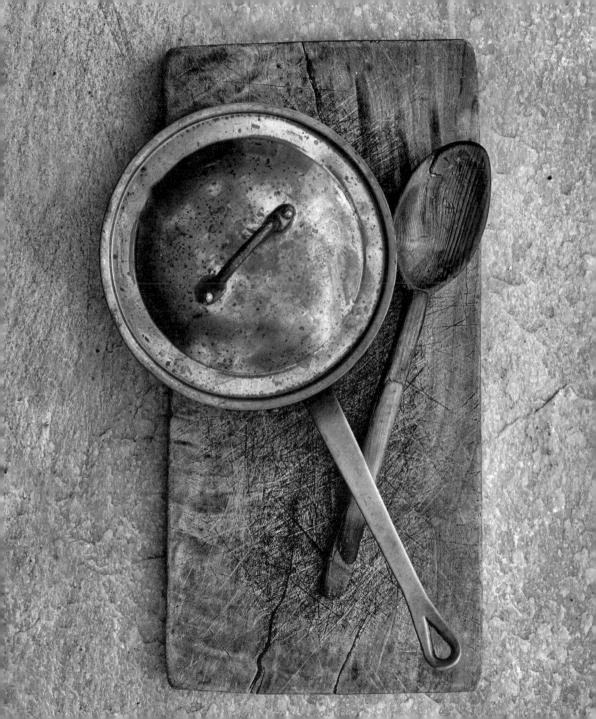

SOUP BASICS

When I first began making my own soups there was a lot of trial and error. If there were mistakes to be made, I probably made them. From the big disasters (almost burning down the kitchen) to the smaller mistakes (forgetting to take out the bay leaf before blending) I have learned quite a bit along the way. So this chapter is dedicated to the Stephen of the past – it includes all the tips, tricks and staples I wish I had known before I started. I have made the errors, so you don't have to.

EQUIPMENT

One of the great things about making soup is that you don't need any special equipment, so you'll probably already have everything you need to get started. If you do need to buy a piece of equipment, such as a liquidiser or blender, buy the best you can afford, because this will save you time and effort during soup preparation. In this section I have put together all the 'essentials' that will help you recreate my soup recipes really easily.

KNIVES
I like to have a small paring knife and a larger knife (for chopping) ready to hand. Buy the best knives you can afford and keep them as sharp as possible. Blunt knives slip off the vegetables easily and can cause accidents. Take care of your knives by washing them carefully in soapy water; never put them in the dishwasher as it blunts them and it's a struggle to get them really sharp again. Remember always to chop and cut vegetables at a slant, moving away from your fingers.

CHOPPING BOARDS
Ideally, use a flexible plastic chopping board. They don't absorb smells, can go in the dishwasher and you can fold the board at the edge after chopping vegetables and tip them directly into the pan, avoiding spills. Wooden boards are great but do need a lot of care and glass boards tend to blunt knives very quickly.

PEELERS
You don't always need to peel the vegetables for our soups, but when you do, use a peeler that you're comfortable with. They come in many shapes and sizes, from side peelers to front peelers, serrated blades and easy-grip handles. We have ended up with several at home because each of us has our own particular favourite.

SCALES
Digital cooking scales will provide the most sensitive weighing mechanism, allowing you to measure accurately to within 1 g or 1 oz.

SPOONS
Measuring spoons are really handy for measuring out ingredients in 'teaspoons' and 'tablespoons'. A good-sized ladle is also invaluable for easily

dishing up generous helpings of soup. A long stirring spoon made of either metal or silicone would be handy, but avoid using wooden spoons as they can absorb flavours, which can then be accidentally transferred from one soup to another.

MEASURING JUGS

Use glass or clear plastic jugs so that you can easily see the liquid level. You will need jugs with a minimum capacity of 1 litre (2 pints).

HAND OR STICK BLENDER

The more powerful the blender, the quicker and more smoothly it will blend the soups. I use a 700W hand blender that has seen me through the development of a multitude of textures, blends and flavours. (Read more about blenders and blending techniques on page 35.)

LIQUIDISER

Any counter-top or jar blender will happily do the job of blending the soups but you do have less control over the texture than you would with a hand blender.

HERB INFUSER OR MUSLIN

An infuser or muslin is necessary for any recipes where herbs or spices have to be put into the soup during the cooking process and then removed before blending or serving.

PANS

The main requirement here is a pan with a heavy-bottomed base that will sit firmly and evenly on the hob. I avoid aluminium as I find it can react with the food and therefore slightly change the

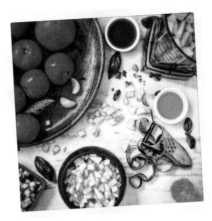

taste. The best options are stainless-steel pans as they work well on all types of hobs.

FREEZER BAGS

The Soupologie soups all freeze really well, so if you do want to cook and store, simply decant any excess soup that you've made into sturdy freezer bags with a good seal (and remember to label them with the recipe name and date!). The soups can be frozen and stored for around three months, ready to defrost and use at any time. When you're ready to use some frozen soup, defrost it slowly in the fridge over a period of 24 hours, rather than zapping it in the microwave. The process of freezing breaks down the cell walls of the vegetables, with the result that when you defrost the soups, the water content from within the vegetables will have separated. By defrosting them slowly, this separation is less apparent and the soups will simply need a good stir when you are heating them up.

COOKING TECHNIQUES

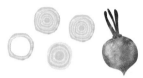

Certain skills and techniques that I have honed over the years have become an integral part of my recipes, which is why I want to share them with you here. None of them are complicated or time-consuming.

CARAMELISING ONIONS

Caramelising is the technique by which vegetables such as onions are slowly cooked in a little oil to enable all the natural sugars from the onions to be released. The onions should be peeled and chopped, but not too finely. Heat the oil in the pan before adding the onions and then keep the heat on medium to low so that the onions sauté gently without burning. As the sugars are released, the onions will change from being opaque in colour to translucent. At this point you need to stir the onions around well, but gently, picking up any brown deposits at the bottom of the pan (these are the caramelised natural sugars). Keep stirring well to avoid burning. The colour of the onions will change from white to golden brown, at which point they are done.

If the onions are under-caramelised, they won't have released as much sugar and the soup will not blend as well as it should; it may also have a slightly 'raw onion' taste to it. If the onions are over-caramelised, they will create a bitter taste – like burnt sugar – and the colour will be dark brown, which will obviously affect the colour of the soup. It's difficult to suggest a precise time for

"If ever I'm asked to supply a head shot of myself, no-one ever knows how close I've come to needing my eyebrows and eyelashes photoshopped into the picture thanks to a near-disaster in the kitchen. Unfortunately I had left oil heating in a pan which I then forgot about. Trust me, when you watch actors on TV and in the movies saving all and sundry amid black smoke and flames, it's not like that in real life. In a split second, the entire kitchen was choking and overwhelmed. So a word of warning: it's not just chip pans that go up in flames; once you've got heat under some oil, never leave it unattended."

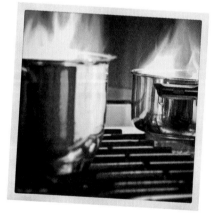

the caramelisation process, as it depends on the strength of your hob, the type of pan you are using, the amount of onions, and so on, but it is likely to be around 8–10 minutes.

BLENDING

I'm a bit passionate about blending! It's the stage in soup-making where you can release the natural creaminess from the vegetables and create a velvety smooth soup. When we do tastings in stores, people often remark that they can't believe my soups don't have cream in them. I never use cream and, as I explain, it's all about the blend. The starting point is that the vegetables must be soft enough to blend. If you can cut through them easily with your stirring spoon, they are ready to be blended. I like to use a stick blender as it means I can blend the soup in the pan without having to transfer it to a jug, and I can move the blender around the pan, clockwise and anti-clockwise, ensuring that every part of the soup is reached.

The time it takes to blend a soup will vary according to the power of the blender, the volume of soup in the pan and the type of vegetable that's being blended. For example, a soup with a high proportion of celery, leeks or kale will be tougher to blend than one with potatoes or broccoli. To achieve a really smooth soup using a 700W hand blender, you will need to blend for around five minutes, then cook the soup for a few more minutes before blending again. By partially blending first, you will be breaking down the vegetables into small particles, so they will soften more quickly and break up more easily in the second round of

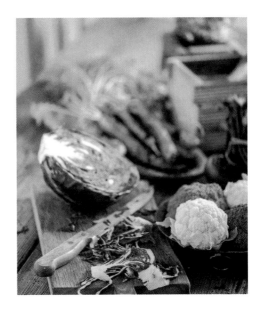

blending. If you prefer more texture to your soups, reduce the blending time to suit your taste.

CHOPPING VEGETABLES

The general rule is that the finer you chop the vegetables, the quicker they will cook. The most important rule, however, is that all the vegetables should be chopped to more or less the same size so that they cook evenly.

PARTIALLY COVERING THE PAN

You'll find that in the instructions to all my recipes I recommend partially covering the pan with the lid. This speeds up the cooking process and also decreases the amount of evaporation that occurs during the cooking process, ensuring that the soups do not become too thick or dried out.

STORE-CUPBOARD ESSENTIALS

There are some ingredients that I always like to use, some that just make life easier and others that give the soups a higher nutritional value. All of the ingredients listed here have a permanent home in my store cupboard.

PINK HIMALAYAN ROCK SALT
This is a pretty, pink salt that has a slightly more subtle flavour than sea salt and ordinary table salt. I like using it in my recipes but I leave the choice entirely up to you, as you need to season to taste. I would caution, though, that despite being rock salt and having more minerals in it than table salt, like all salts, it should be used sparingly.

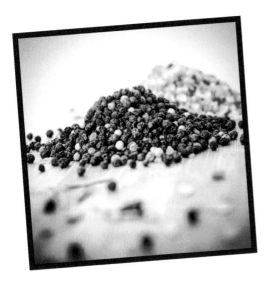

FRESHLY GROUND BLACK PEPPER
My pepper mill is never far away. I tend to leave seasoning my soups until the very end: if you season too early, you don't allow for the natural evaporation that occurs as the soup is cooking and you can end up with a more intense seasoning than you anticipated. Season to taste with both salt and pepper once the soup is blended, and add them gradually, in small amounts. It is difficult to correct seasoning if you overdo it.

GOOD VEGETABLE STOCK
My vegan broth recipe on page 43 can be used as a stock for all the soup recipes in this book that need 'vegetable stock'. Alternatively, you can buy stock in many forms, from fresh to frozen, powdered or cubed, or with certain health features, such as reduced salt, gluten-free, organic ingredients and so on. If you are buying stock, choose the healthiest one available, with the least amount of salt and preservatives (watch out particularly for monosodium glutamate). Some people may prefer to use a meat stock. I always use a vegetable stock with a vegetable soup as I feel that the vegetables should not be overwhelmed by a stock – the idea is to subtly enhance the flavour profile, not drown it out. The use of stock at all is entirely optional; you may prefer to use plain water and just let the natural flavours of the vegetables shine through.

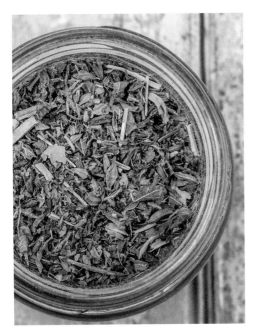

I do prefer rapeseed over olive oil in this instance, as I find that olive oil leaves behind a taste that, for me, interferes with the flavour of the vegetables.

DRIED HERBS

I always like to have a selection of dried herbs for those occasions when fresh ones aren't readily available. You can substitute fresh herbs for dried ones, but remember that dried herbs are up to four times more intense than fresh ones, so you will need to adapt the quantity you use in the soups accordingly.

CANNED TOMATOES

It is so useful to have canned tomatoes in your cupboard – just make sure that the brand you buy is free from added sugar and salt. Check labels and buy tomatoes that are sitting in their own natural juice, without additives.

WILD RICE

A packet of wild rice in the cupboard means that you can always summon up a healthy meal. Wild rice is low in fat and has no cholesterol. It is very versatile and – for some people – it is the ultimate comfort food, making it a perfect addition to any of the soups.

CANNED BEANS

From adzuki to cannellini, pinto to butterbeans, I always have a couple of tins of beans handy as they're all rich in protein, high in fibre and full of minerals and vitamins. Having them in cans, rather than dried, means that they are readily available for adding to soups, casseroles or stews, giving them an immediate nutritional kick.

RAPESEED OIL

Rapeseed oil used to be demonised, with good reason, because it contained large amounts of toxic erucic acid. In the 1950s it was banned for human consumption by the American FDA. However, a cleaned-up version of rapeseed oil emerged in the 1980s and it has become steadily more popular, as it is low in saturated fats and has a higher smoking point than olive oil, making it good for frying and sautéing. It is now grown extensively in many countries and there is also a wonderful assortment of artisanal cold-pressed varieties on offer. I don't think it's necessary to use an expensive cold-pressed oil for the soups, but

SOUPER TOPPERS

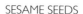

All of my soups taste delicious on their own, but sometimes it's fun to add a topping for additional flavour or texture. Listed here and pictured (right) are some of my favourite soup toppings.

TOASTED COCONUT FLAKES
These delicious flakes add texture, fun and exotic elegance to most soups. For maximum absorption of their iron, eat with a soup that is rich in Vitamin C, such as our Mulligatawny (page 70) or Spicy Tomato and Red Pepper (page 82). To toast your own, bake them in a low oven (150°C/300°F/Gas Mark 2) for 8–10 minutes until golden brown.

POPPED AMARANTH
Amaranth is a wonderful ingredient for pumping up the protein content of your meal. You can buy it ready-popped from health-food shops or you can prepare your own. Simply heat a heavy-based frying pan – no oil needed – then add a couple of tablespoons of amaranth. It will begin to pop in a couple of seconds. Tip it into a cool dish immediately to prevent burning.

ROASTED SWEETCORN
This is simple and delicious. Put some fresh or canned corn kernels on a baking tray, sprinkle with paprika and ground black pepper, and place in a hot oven (220°C/425°F/Gas Mark 7). Cook for around 15 minutes. Popped corn (popcorn) is a great soup toppper too.

SESAME SEEDS
Sesame seeds are a fantastic source of essential vitamins and minerals, so it's no wonder they have been linked to anti-inflammatory properties as well as metabolic function and oral health. To toast for use as a topping, sprinkle into a dry pan and cook over a medium heat for 3–4 minutes.

HEMP SEED HEARTS
Hemp seeds are full of plant protein, but a bit tough. However, if you buy them shelled, exposing the 'heart', you'll find them really delicious. They are thought to be hunger suppressants, so a great choice if you are trying to shift a little weight.

TOASTED PUMPKIN SEEDS
These nutty seeds are high in zinc, so if you are suffering from a cold, they are an excellent option for helping your immune system. Buy them toasted or toast as for sesame seeds (above).

CHIA SEEDS
These tiny seeds pack a big punch when it comes to nutrition. As you sprinkle them onto the soup, they'll quickly swell up and soften as they absorb the liquid. If you stir them in to thinner soups they will act as a great natural thickener.

SUNFLOWER SEEDS
High in Vitamin E, sunflower seeds are great for skin health. They are delicious to snack on and work perfectly sprinkled on our soups.

FLAXSEEDS

Flaxseeds really are considered a 'souper' food and they are currently the subject of clinical studies that aim to fully substantiate all their health benefits. To unlock their goodness, it is best to partially grind or crush them (or buy them already milled) so your body can digest them easily.

CASHEW CREAM

A cashew-cream swirl on top of a soup is a beautiful way to brighten up the dish. Soak the cashews overnight, then drain and blend with fresh water, a little garlic and a squeeze of lemon. Not only does it add a luxurious extra level to your soup, it also adds valuable protein.

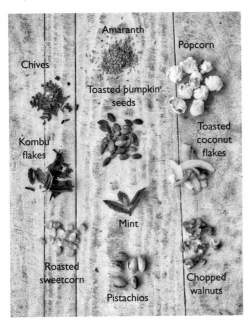

Amaranth

Popcorn

Chives

Toasted pumpkin seeds

Toasted coconut flakes

Kombu flakes

Mint

Roasted sweetcorn

Chopped walnuts

Pistachios

TOFU

Inspired by the classic miso soup, we believe tofu is a great topping option! Whether it is silken and soft, or oven-baked and chewy, tofu adds protein to make that bowl of soup a 'souper-healthy' meal.

ACTIVATED SPROUTS

Try sprouting your toppers! By soaking dry grains, seeds and nuts, you encourage enzymes in them to break down certain molecules that are difficult for the body to absorb. Once this has happened, you can dehydrate them again for a crunchy topping, knowing all the goodness is more accessible to your body. The other option is to continue to let them grow for a few days, and eat them as sprouts. Either way is delicious and nutritious.

QUINOA

Popped or boiled, quinoa has become incredibly popular because it is loaded with important nutrients from protein to minerals, such as manganese. It does not have a strong flavour but adds texture and nutritional value.

CRUMBLED RICE CRACKERS

Crunchy rice crackers are a great gluten-free snack food. Why not use them as an alternative to croutons? Crumbled on top, they add bulk to the soup, helping keep you full and satisfied.

CRUSHED NUTS

Walnuts, pecans, almonds, pistachios and peanuts can enhance the flavour of soups and will add a contrasting crunch. They are also full of healthy fats, fibre and protein. So go nutty and garnish your soups with them on a regular basis.

CHOOSING YOUR SOUP

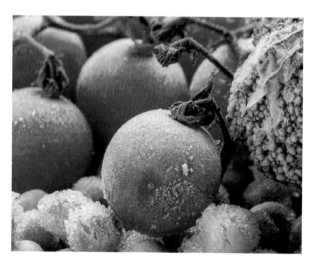

The wide variety of vegetables and fruits in this collection of soup recipes provides you with a glorious edible rainbow, which is why I have organised the soups into colour ranges, creating my very own soup palette. The medical community considers it important for us to eat a balanced diet consisting of different coloured whole foods so as to ensure our bodies absorb a good combination of essential vitamins and minerals. When thinking about those 'five portions of fruit and vegetables a day', as recommended by dietitians and governments around the globe, bear in mind that ideally this should be made up of five different types of fruit and vegetables. Most of my soup

recipes will provide you with two of your five-a-day per serving; having two or more soups in a day will get you well on your way to helping your body receive many of the essential nutrients it needs.

UNDERSTANDING RECIPE ICONS

As each soup has particular nutritional properties that form part of a healthy diet and lifestyle, I thought it would be helpful to create icons so that you can see at a glance the nutritional highlights of each individual soup (see right). These may help you decide which soup to cook when you are having difficulties making up your mind.

"Many of the vegetables that I use can be bought frozen and already prepared. I'm not averse to using frozen veg; in fact, it can often be more nutritious than so-called 'fresh' vegetables that have clocked up hundreds of air miles before landing on your supermarket shelf. If buying and using frozen veggies will encourage you to make these soups and eat more healthily, go for it."

Cleansing

This icon appears next to all the soups that are in our cleansing plans because they contain a variety of different veggies that provide you with as wide a range of nutrients as possible. This includes lots of cruciferous veg (the cabbage family), B vitamins and fibre, as these may all help with the body's natural detoxing process.

Fuller for longer

These soups are the best at filling you up and ensuring you don't crash a few hours later. The magic comes from the combo of fibre, complex carbs, protein and healthy fats, which slows down digestion and absorption. This gives you that lovely comforting, long-lasting feeling of satiety.

Energising

These soups are great when you need a little boost. If you're feeling tired or fatigued, look out for the recipes with this sign. These soups contain naturally occurring carbohydrates and sugars, in combination with fibre. This gives you a steady release of energy, avoiding blood-sugar spikes and falls – keeping you good to go, go, go!

Immune-boosting

These soups may be particularly helpful at the time of year when it seems that everyone has a sniffle or the first pang of a sore throat. You'll find the selection of soups with this icon feature vegetables that are good sources of vitamins C, A and B6, zinc and folic acid, all of which can contribute to the normal function of the immune system and the body's inflammatory responses.

Protein

This icon shows which soups contain a hit of protein. Unlike fat and carbohydrate, protein cannot be stored in the body, so it is very important you ensure you are eating enough.

Skin, hair and nails

Soups with this icon contain hydrating ingredients and lots of vitamins A, C or E. Vitamin C is important for collagen production and counteracting ageing free radicals. Vitamin A helps with water retention and hydration and Vitamin E is great for protecting and repairing your skin and hair.

Stress-busting

These soups contain nutrients such as potassium, magnesium and vitamins B and C. Potassium contributes to the normal function of the nervous system and blood pressure; Vitamin C is important for keeping adrenal glands, which are responsible for the production of stress hormones, healthy. Magnesium can help to relax muscles and reduce anxiety, and Vitamin B helps provide the body with energy after a period of stress.

BROTH BASICS

All the rage for the past few years, broths are back in a big way – but why? What are they good for? The answer is 'pretty much everything', because they are so versatile that you can turn them into innumerable brilliant dishes once you know the hard part, which lies in getting those deep and delicious flavours. Here is my recipe for the perfect vegan broth, and a few of my favourite ways to honour and enrich it.

HOT DRINK REPLACEMENT

I believe sipping on broth throughout the day is far more comforting than tea or coffee. Hot and steaming, brimming with nutrients, it soothes and restores me. Sipping on it throughout the day is also a great way to satisfy your savoury cravings without snacking. You'll see that I have recommended this as part of the souping plans.

NOODLE SOUP

My broth is very easy to turn into a delicious noodle soup. Simply add vegetables chopped into small matchsticks and a few rice noodles (sea spaghetti or kelp noodles make a great alternative). You could also include sesame seeds or tofu to boost the protein content.

RISOTTO

You can use this broth as a substitute for stock in an indulgent risotto. The depth of flavour in the broth will automatically turn your risotto into a delicious dish. In fact, this broth is a great replacement for stock in many recipes.

CASSOULET

Why not try a veggie take on the Provençal classic? Bake root vegetables and haricot beans in this broth with a dash of mustard, thyme and garlic cloves for a truly delightful meal.

GRAVY

Homemade veggie gravy often lacks the depth of the meatier varieties, due to the absence of meat juices, but the rich taste of this broth makes it a perfect base for a vegetable gravy. To make the gravy, caramelise some onions (see page 34), garlic and any herbs you might fancy, until you have a sticky paste. Slowly stir in some chickpea flour (a good gluten-free option) to make a roux, then gradually add the broth, little by little, stirring steadily until you reach the desired thickness.

FREEZE FOR FUTURE USE

This broth is such a useful thing to have on hand that it's worth making more than you need and freezing some for later use. Allow the broth to cool, then pour into labelled, sealable freezer bags or rigid containers and freeze immediately. Remember to allow for expansion, because liquids increase in mass as they freeze. This broth can be stored for 2–3 months. To use, defrost the broth overnight in the fridge, then gently heat in a pan.

If you use this broth as vegetable stock for the recipes in this book, you'll find that its rich umami flavour adds a depth that is rare in vegetarian food. The long ingredient list provides a wonderfully broad selection of nutrients, including vitamins A, B and C, while turmeric's anti-inflammatory properties make this a soothing, restorative broth.

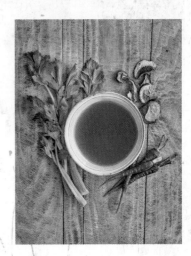

VEGAN BROTH

Makes: 2.5 litres

2 tbsp rapeseed oil

2 large onions, chopped

2 carrots, peeled and chopped

2 celery sticks, trimmed and chopped

1 leek, trimmed and chopped

3 garlic cloves, peeled and chopped

15 g (½ oz) fresh parsley, chopped

1 bay leaf

1 tsp fresh thyme

¼ tsp mustard powder

¼ tsp ground nutmeg

¼ tsp ground turmeric

1 tbsp tomato purée

½ tsp dried kombu flakes

15 g (½ oz) dried porcini mushrooms

Salt and freshly ground black pepper

Caramelise the onions in the oil until they are golden brown (see page 34).

Add the carrots, celery and leek and continue to cook on a low heat for 4–5 minutes.

Add the garlic and cook for a further 1–2 minutes, then add the parsley, bay leaf, thyme, mustard, nutmeg and turmeric.

Cook for 1–2 minutes. Add the tomato purée and stir well.

Add 2.5 litres (4½ pints) water and bring to the boil. Turn down the heat and simmer gently, partially covered, for 35–40 minutes, stirring occasionally.

Add the kombu flakes and the dried mushrooms, and continue to simmer, partially covered for another 15–20 minutes. Season to taste and take off the heat.

Line a sieve or colander with a muslin cloth, some kitchen paper or a coffee filter. Pour the soup through the lined sieve to leave a clear broth.

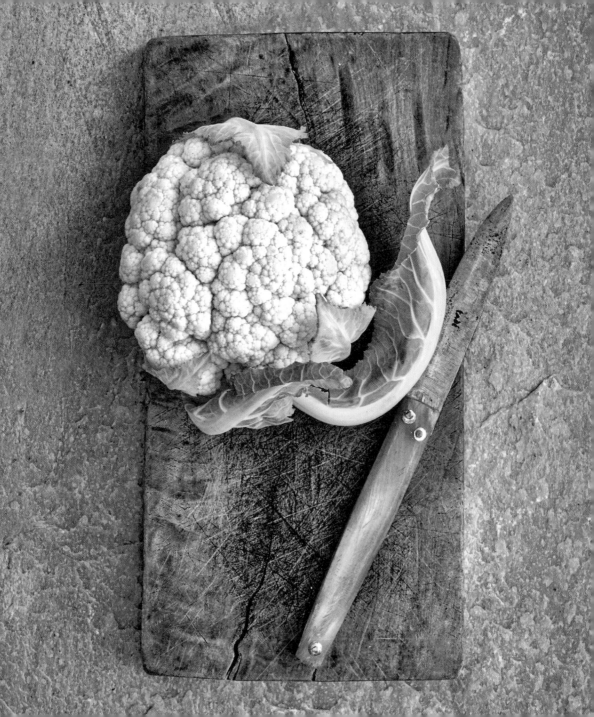

THE WHITE SOUPS

White foods such as bread, pasta and rice get a bad rap because they are often heavily processed before they end up in our cupboards. However, there are lots of super, naturally white vegetables that are full of goodness and nutrients. From trendy cauliflowers and sweet leeks to humble potatoes and onions, I love the variety of textures and creaminess of my white soup collection. From cool Cucumber and Apple to comforting Celeriac and Walnut, I promise you won't get bored with my white soups, which come with the added bonus of health-giving vitamins and minerals.

Jerusalem artichoke is a very under-used vegetable, which may be due to the fact that it is difficult to peel or because it causes a strange and unpredictable reaction in the gut of some people. If you've never had it before, try a small taster of this soup before demolishing a full bowl! The reason this soup merits inclusion in this healthy selection is its inulin content. Not to be confused with insulin, inulin is a sweet, starchy, fibrous substance that goes through the digestive system intact, and on arrival in the colon, contributes to the growth of healthy bacteria. It's this bacterial activity that can create gas in the system and cause discomfort. However, if you have no problem with it, the vegetable is a wonderful source of dietary fibre, potassium, iron and copper.

JERUSALEM ARTICHOKE

Serves 4

2 tbsp rapeseed oil

1 medium onion, chopped

400 g (14 oz) Jerusalem artichokes, peeled and chopped

1 medium carrot, peeled and chopped

1 small leek, trimmed and chopped

1½ sage leaves, chopped

750 ml (1¼ pints) vegetable stock

Salt and freshly ground black pepper

Caramelise the onion in the oil (see *page 34*).

Add the artichoke, carrot, leek and sage. Sweat the vegetables by cooking them on a medium heat, covered, for around 10 minutes, until the vegetables are tender and starting to soften.

Add the vegetable stock and bring to the boil. Then lower the heat and simmer, partially covered, for about 20 minutes, until the vegetables are soft. Stir occasionally.

When cooked, take off the heat and blend until smooth. Season to taste.

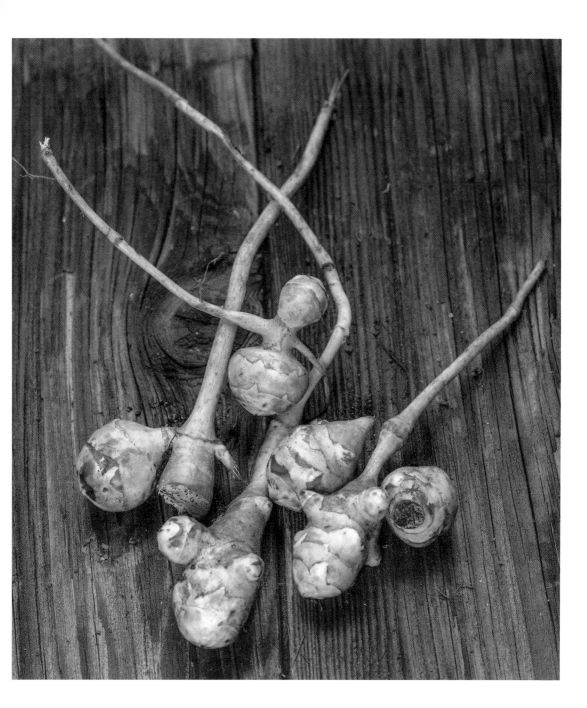

I know it's difficult to move on from associating cauliflower with that horrible smell of boiled, over-cooked cauliflower that wafted through the school dining hall, but trust me, this is cauliflower like you've never had it before. This cruciferous vegetable has recently become incredibly popular as its health benefits are starting to be widely recognised. It is an excellent source of vitamin C and antioxidants and it also contains Vitamin K, which means it is good for bones. It is truly delicious as long as you don't let it cook for too long. The addition of mustard seed turns this milky, creamy vegetable blend into a sensationally tangy treat. Buy the cleanest wholegrain mustard you can, as a lot of the brands include unnecessary sugar. You can use the inner leaves of the cauliflower along with the florets, and you won't need to cook or blend for too long, as this vegetable breaks down very quickly.

CAULIFLOWER AND MUSTARD SEED

Serves 4–6

1 cauliflower, washed, trimmed and diced

3½ tbsp rapeseed oil

2 large onions, peeled and diced

3 strips lemon zest

2 tsp wholegrain mustard

1.1 litre (1¾ pints) vegetable stock

Salt and freshly ground black pepper

Roast the cauliflower in a hot oven (220°C/425°F/Gas Mark 7) for 30 minutes, until the edges just begin to turn golden.

Caramelise the onion in the oil for 5–10 minutes (*see page 34*).

Add the cauliflower and lemon zest to the onion. Cook on a medium to low heat for another 2–3 minutes.

Add the wholegrain mustard, followed by the vegetable stock and bring to the boil. Turn down the heat and simmer for around 8–10 minutes, until the cauliflower is completely soft.

Take the soup off the heat and carefully remove the lemon zest. Blend until completely smooth and season to taste.

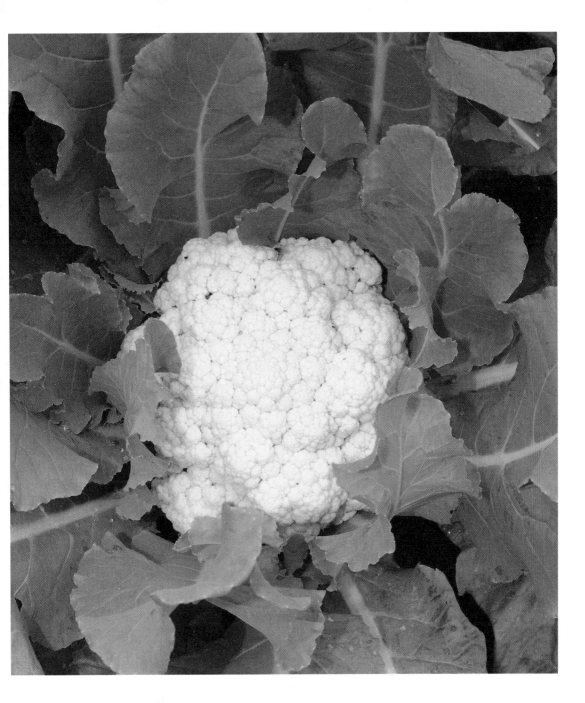

Celeriac is unprepossessing in appearance and tough to peel, but it's worthwhile persevering with this root vegetable, because underneath all that hard skin is a beautifully nutty, creamy vegetable that is versatile, healthy and delicious. You can use it in so many ways, from being an alternative to mashed potatoes to an alternative to spaghetti – it produces brilliant results from a spiralizer. It's also a great ingredient for a soup, as you'll find out, and the strong flavour is perfectly complemented by a drizzle of walnut oil. Nutritionally celeriac has it all going on: it's low in calories and is a good source of fibre, thiamin and Vitamin C. So unearth that inner celeriac and get cooking!

CELERIAC AND WALNUT

Serves 6

2 tbsp rapeseed oil

1 large onion, peeled and diced

1 leek, trimmed and chopped

1 celeriac, peeled and diced

1 potato, peeled and chopped

2 garlic cloves, peeled and finely chopped

2 celery sticks, trimmed and chopped

1.5 litres (2¾ pints) vegetable stock

½ eating apple, unpeeled, cored and chopped

Salt and freshly ground black pepper

Walnut oil for drizzling

Caramelise the onion in the oil (*see page 34*).

Add the leek, celeriac, potato, garlic and celery. Cook, partially covered, on a medium heat, stirring occasionally, for around 20 minutes, until the vegetables are tender and starting to soften.

Add the vegetable stock and bring to the boil. Once boiling, reduce the heat and simmer, partially covered, for a further 10–15 minutes, until all the vegetables are soft.

Add the apple, stir and cook for a further minute, then take off the heat and blend until the soup is smooth. Season with salt and pepper to taste. Serve with a swirl of walnut oil, and add a few walnut halves on the top for texture, if you like.

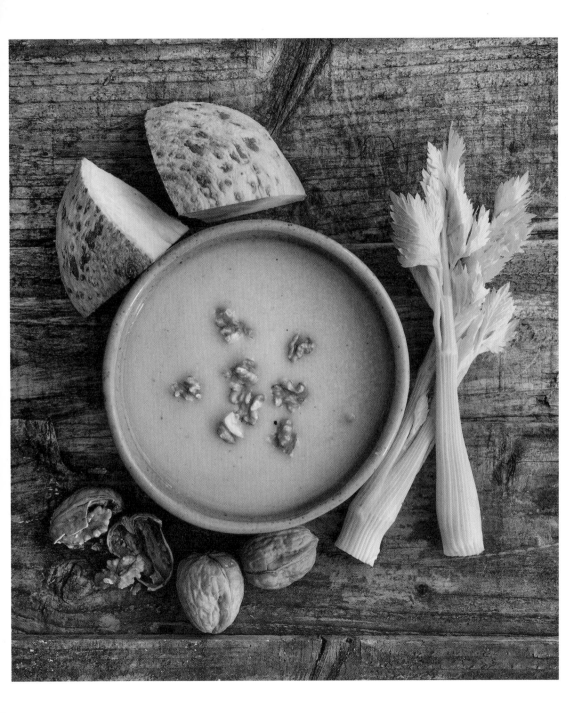

This is a light, fragrant soup that is naturally sweetened by apples. When blended really well, it has a deliciously creamy texture. If you don't often eat parsnips, they're worth reconsidering: they are easy to peel, readily available and have a distinctive flavour that works well with fruit. I've made parsnip and pear soup on many occasions, and even added in cranberries; the parsnip seems to happily accept them all, becoming sweeter or more piquant accordingly. Parsnips have great nutritional benefits too, as they yield lots of Vitamin C, fibre and folic acid, but you'll want to enjoy this for the taste and texture. For a real treat, top with roasted parsnip crisps; simply brush some thin slices with olive oil, roast in a medium oven for around 30 minutes, turning them once, and then float them on top of the soup.

PARSNIP AND APPLE

Serves 4–5

2 tbsp rapeseed oil

1 medium onion, chopped

1 kg (2¼ lb) parsnips, peeled and chopped

1 leek, finely sliced

1 celery stick, chopped

1 bay leaf

1.5 litres (2¾ pints) vegetable stock

1 eating apple, cored but unpeeled

Salt and freshly ground black pepper

Caramelise the onion in the oil (*see page 34*). Add the parsnip, leek, celery and bay leaf and let the vegetables sweat for 5–6 minutes, partially covered. Stir occasionally.

Add the vegetable stock and bring to the boil, then turn down the heat and simmer gently, partially covered, for around 10 minutes, until the parsnips are soft. Give it an occasional stir.

Remove the bay leaf and discard. Add the apple and cook for a further 1–2 minutes.

Take off the heat and blend the soup until completely smooth. Season to taste.

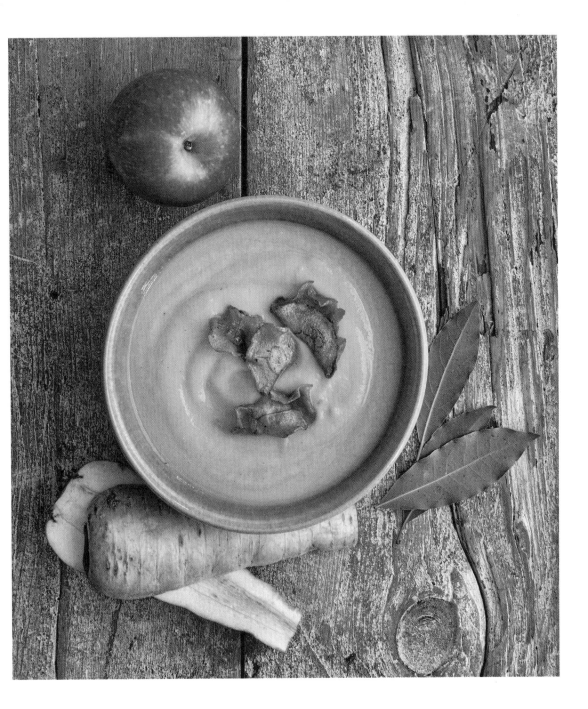

This delicate soup, laced with barely wilted greenery, works perfectly to combine starchy carbohydrates with super-nutritious dark green leaves that are dropped into the soup at the last minute. Aim for 60 g (2 oz) of green leaves in total, which may be a mixture of watercress, spinach and rocket (as here), or just one or two types of leaves. Choose potatoes that aren't waxy, as you want them to easily disintegrate into fluffiness once cooked. Having experimented with several different types over the years, my preference is to use either King Edward or Maris Piper potatoes, where possible. Toasted sesame seeds (*see page 38*) sprinkled over the top work wonderfully as a quick nutritional boost and create added texture.

POTATO AND SUMMER LEAVES

Serves 4

2 tbsp rapeseed oil

1 large onion, peeled and diced

3 medium potatoes, peeled and diced

½ tsp ground nutmeg

½ tsp mustard powder

630 ml (21 fl oz) vegetable stock

20 g (¾ oz) watercress

20 g (¾ oz) spinach

20 g (¾ oz) rocket

Salt and freshly ground black pepper

Caramelise the onion in the oil (*see page 34*) for 3–4 minutes.

Add the potatoes and cook on a medium to low heat for around 20 minutes, until the potatoes are tender.

Add the nutmeg and mustard to the potatoes, followed by the vegetable stock. Bring to the boil, then lower the heat and simmer for 5–10 minutes, until the potatoes are soft.

Take off the heat and blend until completely smooth.

Drop the watercress, spinach and rocket leaves into the soup and stir in well, letting the heat of the soup wilt them. Season to taste and serve, making sure that everyone gets a good portion of leaves.

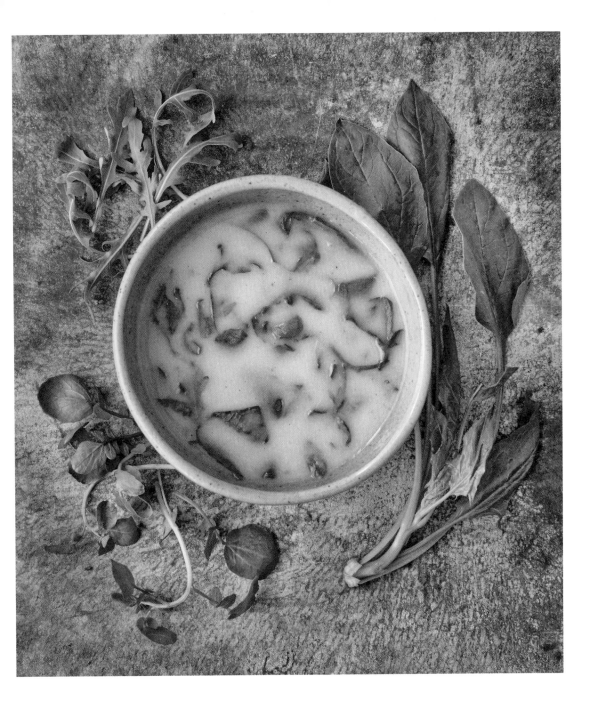

Fruit soups are popular in Scandinavian countries and I can heartily recommend them. Full of fruit and vegetables, including all their flesh, pulp and fibre, these soups ensure that you don't just get the sugar from the fruit, like a juice, but the whole food. This is hugely beneficial, because the fibre acts to slow down the rate at which your body absorbs the fructose (fruit sugar) and so ensures you don't have an energy spike followed by an energy crash. This fruit soup combines those English staples – apples and cucumbers – accompanied by tropical indulgent coconut, to make a smooth and creamy delight. If you have pink Himalayan rock salt in your store cupboard, this adds a subtle difference to the taste, and increases the mineral content of the soup.

CUCUMBER AND APPLE

Serves 8

1 tbsp coconut oil

2 shallots, chopped

2 large cucumbers, peeled and chopped

375 ml (13 fl oz) vegetable stock

115 g (4 oz) seedless white grapes

2 eating apples, peeled, cored and chopped

3 fresh mint leaves

250 ml (8½ fl oz) coconut yoghurt

Pinch of rock salt

Ground black pepper

Maple syrup (optional)

Caramelise the shallot following the method for caramelising onions (see page 34).

Allow the shallot to cool, then add all the remaining ingredients and blend until smooth.

If desired, add maple syrup to taste. Cover and chill in the fridge for 3–4 hours. Serve with a pretty mint leaf on the top.

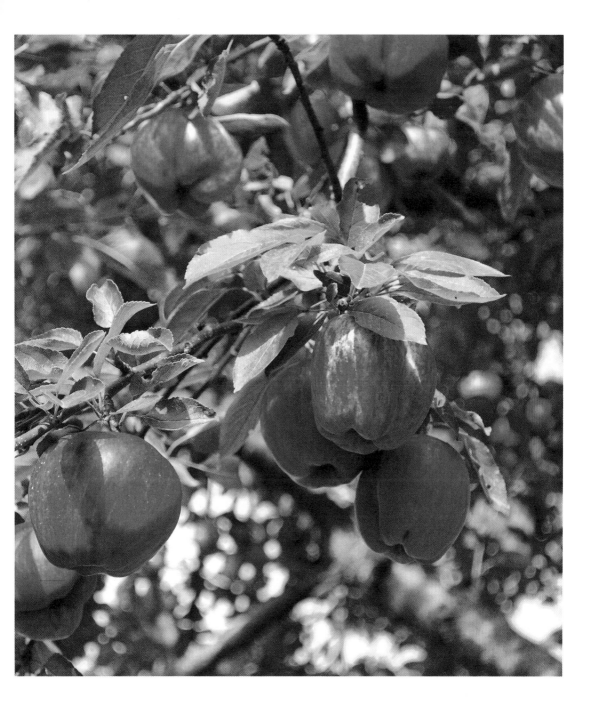

Apples and pears are most commonly used in desserts. This is, of course, because they are naturally sweet, due to the fructose they contain. However, while I love a good apple and pear crumble as much as the next person, I have discovered that these two fruits work exceptionally well with savoury flavours too. And when you add herbs and spices, like the sage, ginger and parsley used here, you can bring out notes in the apple and pear that will really surprise you. The underlying vegetable stock also tones down the sweetness of the fruit, so it becomes quite subtle. This soup is delicious chilled, but it is even better served piping hot in the cooler months, when it can help you fight colds and other germs, as the apples and pears are fibre-rich and full of vitamins. Additionally, anti-inflammatory ginger is really good at helping blocked noses and soothing sore throats.

APPLE AND PEAR

Serves 4–5

2 tbsp rapeseed oil

1 cooking apple, peeled and cored

3 eating apples, peeled and cored

3 pears, peeled and cored

2 sage leaves, finely chopped

1 bay leaf

7.5g (¼ oz) grated fresh ginger

1.25 litres (2 pints) vegetable stock

1 tbsp finely chopped parsley

Freshly ground black pepper

Maple syrup (optional)

Heat the oil in a pan and add the apple and pear, along with the sage, bay leaf and ginger. Let the mixture sweat for 5–6 minutes, partially covered. Stir occasionally.

Add the vegetable stock, stir well and bring to the boil. Then turn down the heat and simmer gently, for 2–3 minutes, stirring occasionally.

Take off the heat, add the parsley and blend the soup until completely smooth. Season to taste with black pepper and, if it tastes slightly too tart for you, add a little maple syrup.

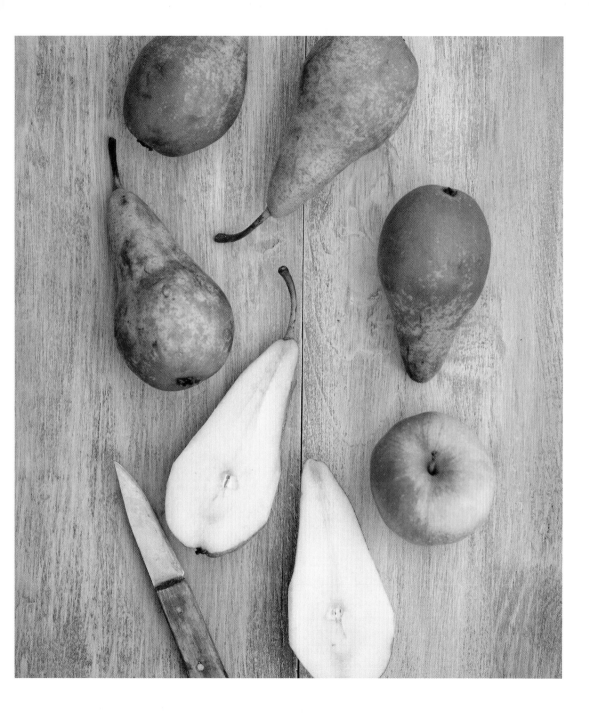

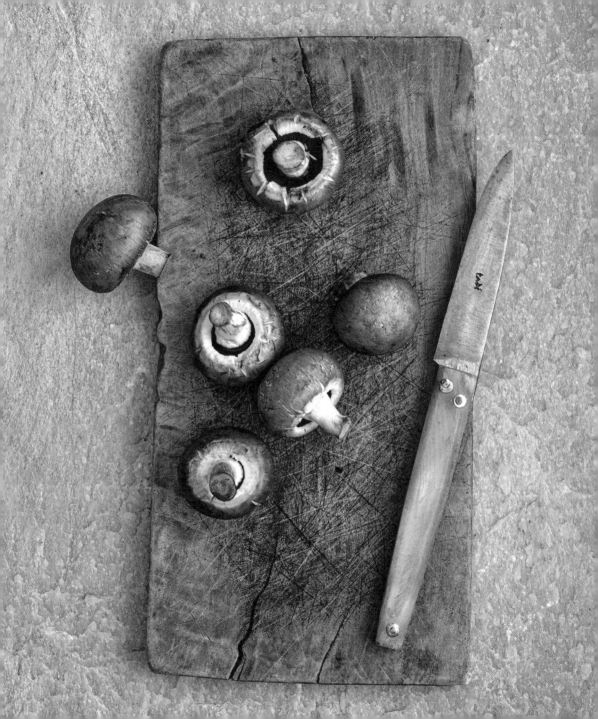

THE BROWN SOUPS

Mixing vegetables of varying colours often results in a brown-coloured soup, so the beauty of brown means that you're getting a rainbow of benefits in one fell swoop (or one fell 'soup' even!). My brown collection is a great option for when you're feeling in need of an overall health kick. Try my Mushroom Soup for cloudy days when your Vitamin D may be running low, dive into Miso or Mulligatawny when you're feeling cosmopolitan, and serve the London Particular to guests looking for a British classic.

The pungent aroma of garlic roasting gently in the oven is one of my favourite smells. It takes me back to when I first started Soupologie; each week the amount of garlic I was roasting grew exponentially, until it outgrew the kitchen completely! Studies have shown that garlic is associated with improved blood circulation, and the strong yet sweet flavour of this soup should enable you to reduce the amount of added salt you need, which will also be helpful for your blood pressure.

ROASTED GARLIC SOUP

Serves 3–4

For the roasted garlic
2 garlic bulbs (about 25 cloves, unpeeled)
1 tbsp rapeseed oil
Salt and freshly ground black pepper

For the remainder of the soup
2 tbsp rapeseed oil
1 large onion, chopped
1½ tsp chopped fresh thyme
15 garlic cloves, peeled and chopped
850 ml (1½ pints) vegetable stock
Salt and freshly ground black pepper
Garlic oil (optional)

Pre-heat the oven to 190°C/375°F/Gas Mark 5.

To roast the garlic: separate the two garlic bulbs into cloves. Place them unpeeled in an ovenproof bowl and add the oil, a pinch of salt and a little black pepper. Mix together so that all the garlic cloves are well covered in oil. Tightly seal the bowl with silver foil and roast for 40–45 minutes. Allow to cool, then squeeze out the flesh from each clove, discarding the skins.

To make the soup: caramelise the onion (see page 34) in the oil until golden brown. Add the thyme and the raw chopped garlic and continue to cook on a low heat for 3–4 minutes.

Add the roasted garlic, followed by the vegetable stock. Stir and bring to the boil. Turn down the heat and simmer gently, partially covered, for about 5–6 minutes, stirring occasionally.

Take off the heat and blend the soup until completely smooth. Season to taste. Drizzle a little garlic oil over the top for an even richer flavour.

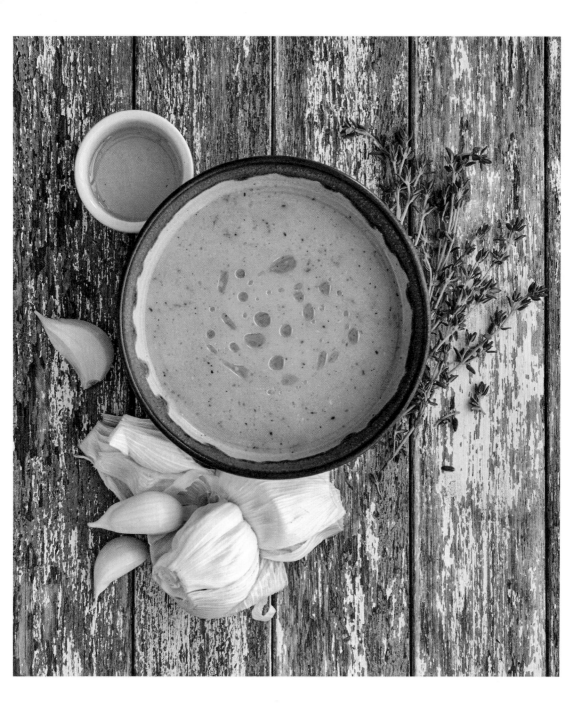

We love lentils at Soupologie, so I decided to go the distance and create a soup that contains three different types of this pulse. It also contains flavoursome vegetables and some Indian-sourced spices, such as cinnamon and cayenne pepper, turning this almost into a traditional daal. Naturally, the three stars of this recipe are the red, green and beluga lentils, all of which contribute their own flavours. The dash of lime juice sharpens the taste, but don't overdo it or it may completely overwhelm the subtlety of the soup. This soup is great if you're feeling under the weather or suffering from poor digestion: the lentils are fantastic for maintaining good gut health. If you like, add some flat parsley on top for extra vitamins.

THREE-LENTIL SOUP

Serves 5–6

2 tbsp rapeseed oil

1 large onion, chopped

4 garlic cloves, peeled and chopped

2 celery sticks, trimmed and chopped

½ tsp ground coriander seed

1 tsp turmeric

¼ tsp cinnamon

¼ tsp cayenne pepper

90 g (3¼ oz) dried split red lentils

45 g (1½ oz) ready-cooked (canned or vac-packed) beluga lentils

90 g (3¼ oz) dried green lentils

1.5 litres (2¾ pints) vegetable stock

1½ tsp fresh lime juice

Salt and freshly ground black pepper

Caramelise the onion in the oil (*see page 34*).

Add the garlic, celery, coriander seed, turmeric, cinnamon and cayenne pepper and let the mixture sweat for 5–6 minutes, partially covered. Stir occasionally.

Wash and drain the lentils, then mix in well. Add the vegetable stock, stir well and bring to the boil.

Turn down the heat and simmer gently until the lentils are completely cooked. Stir regularly to make sure the lentils do not stick to the bottom of the pan.

Add the lime juice and stir in well.

Take off the heat and blend the soup until completely smooth. Season to taste.

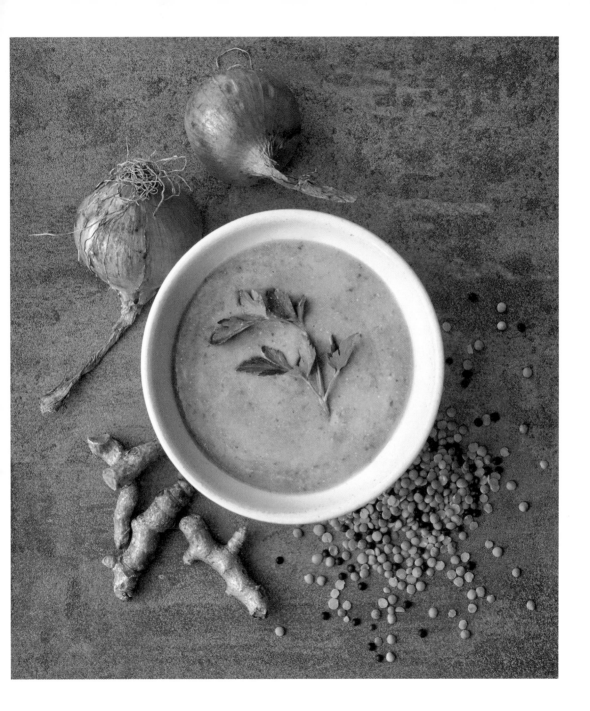

This recipe harks back to the days when London – in particular – was engulfed in smog, or 'pea-soupers', because of coal and wood burning fires. This thick, dense soup, which is traditionally made with ham hock and peas, was an edible representation of the foggy city. You'll see that I have removed the ham but have nevertheless created a meaty-tasting soup from yellow split peas, for a deliciously warming soup that provides protein and fibre.

LONDON PARTICULAR

Serves 4

125 g (4½ oz) dried yellow split peas

2 tbsp rapeseed oil

1 small onion, peeled and diced

1 carrot, peeled and diced

1 celery stick, washed, trimmed and diced

1 bay leaf

3 sprigs thyme

125 g (4½ oz) frozen peas

¾ tsp nutmeg

¾ tsp mustard powder

900 ml (1½ pints) vegetable stock

Salt and freshly ground black pepper

Wash and drain the yellow split peas then put them into a microwave-safe bowl with a lid, and add 500 ml (16 fl oz) water. Cook in the microwave on high power for 10–12 minutes until the peas have started to swell and absorb water. Check and stir them every 2 minutes, adding extra water if needed. The peas don't need to be completely cooked, just softened. Drain when cooked.

On the hob, caramelise the onion in the oil for 2–3 minutes (see page 34). Add the cooked split peas, carrot, celery, bay leaf and thyme. Cook for around 20 minutes, partially covered, on a medium to low heat until the vegetables become tender.

Add the peas, nutmeg and mustard powder and stir well, then add the vegetable stock and bring to the boil. Turn down the heat and simmer, partially covered, until the yellow split peas are completely cooked (around 10–15 minutes).

Remove and discard the bay leaf and thyme. Take off the heat, blend the soup until completely smooth and season to taste.

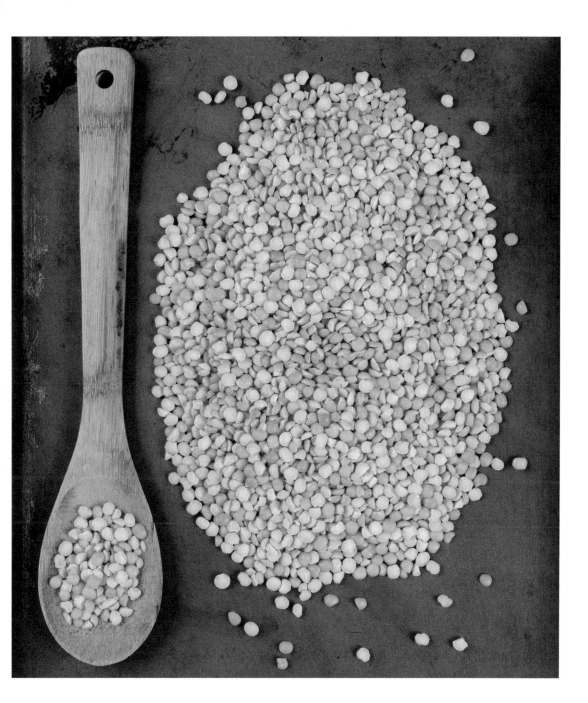

Miso soup is a staple in Japanese cuisine, where it is considered to have important health properties. Outside of Japanese restaurants, it's very hard to find a high-quality miso soup, but in fact it's not very complicated to prepare, as long as you source the right ingredients. The taste of miso is tangy and naturally salty because of the kombu seaweed. This particular recipe can be added to as you wish: mushrooms or noodles (such as soba, rice or buckwheat noodles) work especially well (see the Souper Tip below for more ideas). In this recipe I have suggested the ingredients that I like to complement the base miso flavour.

JAPANESE MISO

Serves 3–4

7 g (¼ oz) kombu flakes

1 tbsp sake

1 tsp brown rice syrup

1.25 cm (½ in) piece fresh root ginger, peeled and finely grated

30 g (1 oz) miso paste

Put 1 litre (1 ¾ pints) water into a pan and add the kombu flakes and sake. Bring to the boil.

Lower the heat to a simmer, add the brown rice syrup and ginger, and stir in well.

Simmer for 4–5 minutes, stirring frequently. Lower the heat and stir in the miso paste until it is fully dissolved.

Souper Tip This soup can be used as the base for a variety of miso soup recipes. Try adding one or more of the following ingredients for added flavour: finely sliced spring onions, finely sliced asparagus spears, cubed silken tofu, dried nori or wakame seaweed, finely chopped Swiss chard, mangetout, mushrooms or noodles.

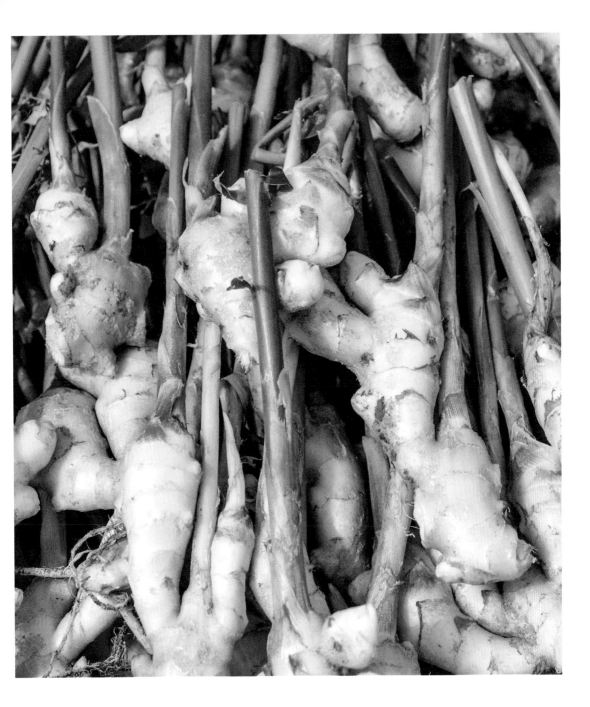

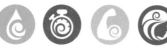

MULLIGATAWNY

Serves 4

For the soup

30 g (1 oz) dried yellow split peas

2 tbsp rapeseed oil

1 small onion, chopped

1 garlic clove, chopped

1 carrot, chopped

2 potatoes, peeled and chopped

1¼ tsp mustard seed

¾ tsp fenugreek seed

1½ tsp ground ginger

50 g (1¾ oz) creamed coconut

133g (4¾ oz) canned chopped tomatoes

2 tbsp tomato purée

650 ml (22 fl oz) vegetable stock

Salt and freshly ground black pepper

For the curry paste

1 tsp rapeseed oil

1 garlic clove, chopped

1 tbsp tomato purée

1 tsp agave nectar

1 tbsp mild curry powder

1 tbsp white wine vinegar

Pinch of salt

Wash and drain the yellow split peas, then place them in a microwave-safe bowl with a lid, together with 130 ml (4¼ fl oz) water. Cook on high power for 10–12 minutes until the peas have started to swell and absorb water. Check and stir every 2 minutes, adding extra water if needed. The peas don't need to be completely cooked, just softened. Drain.

Make the curry paste: put all the curry paste ingredients into a bowl and blend together until you have a smooth paste.

On the hob, caramelise the onion in the oil (*see page 34*).

Add the garlic, carrot, potato and yellow split peas. Stir in well, then add the mustard seed, fenugreek and ginger. Let the vegetables sweat, partially covered, on a medium to low heat for around 20 minutes, until they become tender.

Add the curry paste and creamed coconut. Stir until the coconut has dissolved then pour in the chopped tomatoes and tomato purée, stirring well.

Add the vegetable stock to the soup and bring everything up to the boil. Then turn down the heat and simmer, partially covered, until the yellow split peas are cooked through. This is a chunky soup, so it does not need blending. Season to taste, give everything a good stir, then serve.

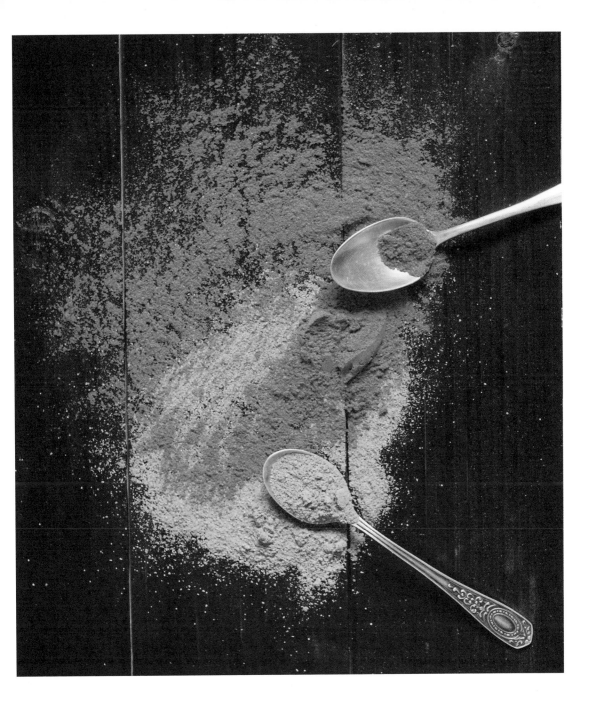

Mushrooms certainly divide opinion, but I'm a great fan – they come in such a rich variety of shapes, sizes, textures and flavours. I love them all! That distinctive umami taste that they have is instantly recognisable and it is also, of course, what creates the division of opinion. It's worthwhile experimenting with the different varieties of mushroom as you'll find that some have a stronger flavour than others, with wild mushrooms also having a particular texture. This creamy recipe mixes some of my favourite mushrooms together into a velvety brown soup that's rich and mellow. There's an interesting way of increasing the health benefits of this soup: if you leave a handful of mushrooms out in the sunshine for around half an hour, they'll absorb sufficient Vitamin D to supply you with your recommended daily dose. You can then use them in the soup and harness the Vitamin D they've soaked up.

MUSHROOM SOUP

Serves 4

2 tbsp rapeseed oil

1 medium onion, chopped

2 garlic cloves, peeled and chopped

150 g (5½ oz) chestnut mushrooms, roughly chopped

150 g (5½ oz) button cup mushrooms, roughly chopped

150 g (5½ oz) Portobello mushrooms, roughly chopped

1 tsp chopped fresh thyme (leaves only, no stalks)

750 ml (1¼ pints) vegetable stock

Salt and freshly ground black pepper

Caramelise the onion in the oil (see page 34), then add the garlic, mushrooms and thyme, keeping back a few leaves of thyme to garnish.

Partially cover the saucepan and cook on a medium heat for around 10 minutes, until the mushrooms are tender.

Add the vegetable stock to the vegetables and bring everything to the boil. Lower the heat and simmer gently, partially covered, for 3–4 minutes, then remove from the heat.

Season to taste and blend until velvety smooth. Serve with a sprinkling of fresh thyme.

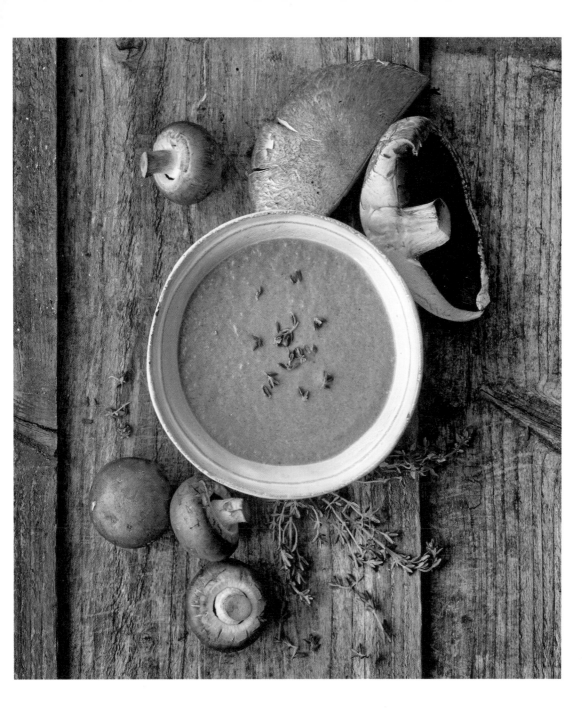

This is a family favourite – the natural aromas and flavours of the onions combine beautifully with the chestnuts and a dash of sweetening agave nectar in this recipe. Chestnuts become deliciously creamy when cooked, delivering the perfect texture. In this recipe, the chestnuts balance the onion; slightly starchy and reasonably high in Vitamin C and low in fat, they are ideal for a healthy diet.

ONION AND CHESTNUT SOUP

Serves 4

2 tbsp rapeseed oil

3 medium–large brown onions, sliced fairly thickly

1 tsp agave nectar

100 g (3½ oz) pre-cooked, vacuum-packed chestnuts

15 g (½ oz) cornflour

1 large garlic clove, peeled and chopped

¼ tsp ground ginger

Salt and freshly ground black pepper

1 litre (1¾ pints) vegetable stock

Heat up the oil in a pan over medium to low heat and add the onions and the agave nectar. Caramelise the onions (see *page 34*) for around 10 minutes, stirring gently until they are a rich golden brown.

While the onions are cooking, chop the chestnuts and prepare the cornflour by adding it to a little cold water in a small bowl. Mix it well until it becomes a smooth paste.

Add the chestnuts, garlic, ginger, and a pinch of salt and pepper to the onion. Stir well and cook, partially covered, over a medium heat for 2–3 minutes.

Pour the vegetable stock into the saucepan and stir well. Then transfer three tablespoons of this mixture into the cornflour paste. Stir really well and then put the entire contents of the bowl into the saucepan.

Bring the soup to the boil stirring constantly, then reduce the heat and let the soup simmer, partially covered, until it starts to thicken, which will take about 3–4 minutes. Stir occasionally.

Take off the heat and blend the soup until completely smooth, adding more seasoning to taste.

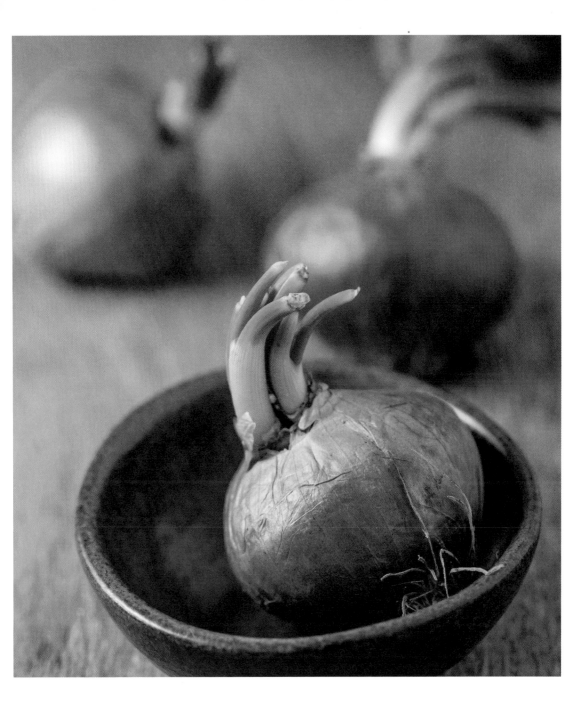

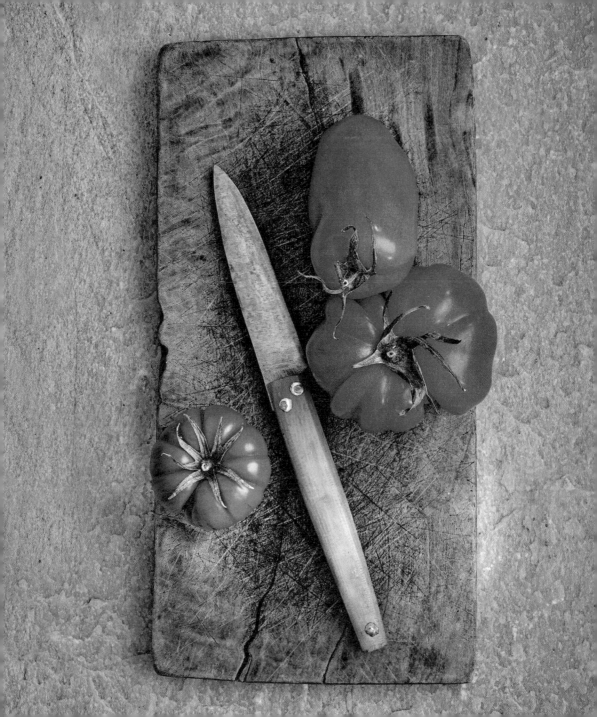

THE RED SOUPS

Lovely lycopene is the reason most of these soups are red. Far from just a pretty pigment, lycopene is a powerful antioxidant which has been put forward for a wide range of medicinal purposes, from sun-ray protection to cancer prevention. And soups are the perfect way to benefit from this natural chemical, which is more easily absorbed when cooked. These red soups are also high in folate, Vitamin C and various flavonoids. Cool off with one of the fruit soups, test how much chilli you can handle in Spicy Tomato and Red Pepper soup, or try my quintessential Tomato and Basil for a delicious new classic.

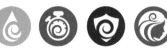

Minestrone, a classic among soups, is so easy – you can just chuck in whatever's lurking at the back of your fridge, right? Well, yes and no; not if you want a great-tasting soup packed with nutrients. This minestrone recipe uses beans and rice to give you a specific range of nutrients, particularly fibre and protein. So by all means use up some of your leftover veggies in this recipe but keep the calories low and nourishment values high with my Soupolo-twist on an everyday minestrone soup.

MINESTRONE

Serves 4–6

2 tbsp rapeseed oil

1 medium onion, chopped

1 large garlic clove, peeled and chopped

2 medium carrots, peeled and chopped

1 leek, washed and chopped

2 celery sticks, trimmed and chopped

1 bay leaf

45 g (1½ oz) dried Arborio risotto rice

220 g (7 ¾ oz) canned cannellini beans

200 g (7 oz) canned chopped plum tomatoes

2 tbsp tomato purée

1 litre (1¾ pints) hot vegetable stock

½ Savoy cabbage, chopped

Salt and freshly ground black pepper

Caramelise the onion in the oil (see *page 34*).

Add the garlic, carrot, leek, celery and bay leaf. Cook on a medium to low heat, with the pan partially covered, sweating the vegetables for around 15 minutes, until they are tender. Stir occasionally.

Drain the cannellini beans. Once the vegetables are soft, add the rice and beans to the vegetables and mix well.

Stir in the chopped tomatoes and tomato purée, then add the hot vegetable stock. Bring everything to the boil, then reduce the heat and simmer gently, with the pan partially covered. Stir occasionally and check on the rice to make sure it is becoming fluffy.

Just before the rice is ready, add the Savoy cabbage and remove the bay leaf. Once the carrots are soft, take off the heat and season to taste. Stir well before serving to make sure you scoop the beans up from the bottom of the pan.

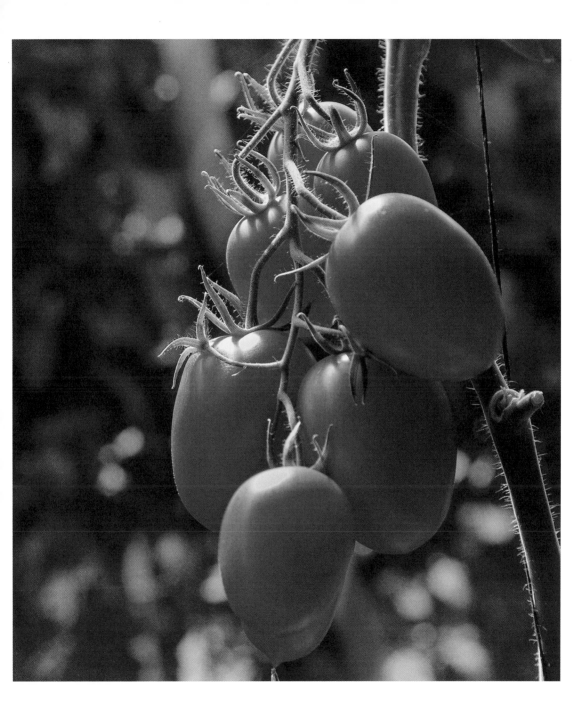

Tomato and basil is a combination that turns up regularly in soups and sauces, but the fresh, homemade version tastes quite different to all the shop-bought varieties. Once you've made this soup for yourself and tasted how delicious it is, you'll find it difficult to go back to the processed varieties (which are often unhealthily high in salt and sugar). I love to rub the fresh basil between my fingers so that its wonderfully aromatic scent lingers. I use this soup endlessly as a base for lots of other dishes, from lasagne to pizzas and risottos. This recipe is pared back and incredibly easy to make, so make loads of it and freeze some so that you know you've always got it to hand. Top with a couple of fresh basil leaves, if you like.

TOMATO AND BASIL

Serves 4–6

2 tbsp rapeseed oil

1 small onion, chopped

1 garlic clove, chopped

1 small carrot, chopped

750 g (26 oz) canned chopped tomatoes

2 tbsp tomato purée

750 ml (1¼ pints) vegetable stock

Small bunch fresh basil, chopped

Salt and freshly ground black pepper

Caramelise the onion in the oil (*see page 34*).

Add the garlic and carrot, then cook on a medium to low heat, with the pan partially covered, for around 10 minutes, until the carrots become tender. Stir occasionally.

Add the tomatoes and tomato purée and stir in well.

Pour in the vegetable stock, and once it has come to the boil, turn down the heat and simmer, partially covered, until the vegetables are soft.

Take off the heat and blend the soup until completely smooth. Add the chopped basil leaves and season to taste. If preferred, blend again briefly, to mix the basil in more finely.

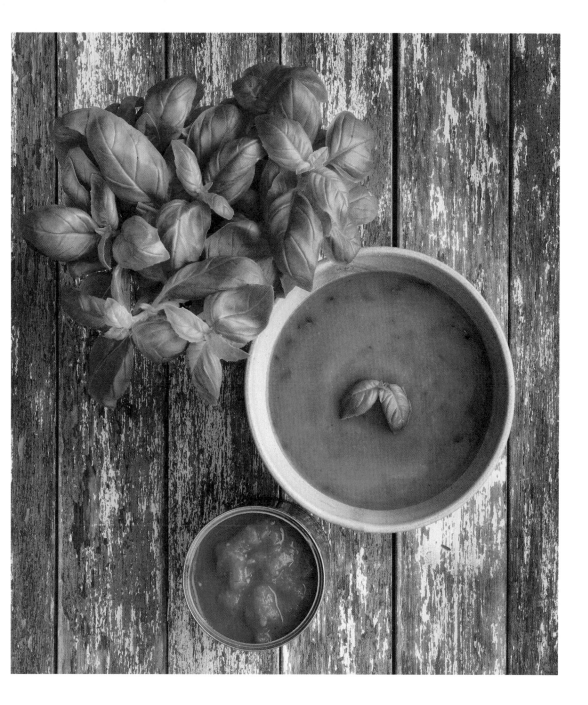

'A tomato soup, and yet so much more than that', is how Giulia's father describes this soup. Giulia is our Office Souperwoman, who works tirelessly on our behalf, trying to organise the numerous post-it notes she finds around the place that are filled with random thoughts and 'important' things we have to do. As such, it seems only fair that she and her family have the chance to try out my hit soups (it's my long-suffering family that have to deal with the misses!). This soup has a real kick to it, with the red pepper bringing a delicious depth of flavour. Nutritionists talk about incorporating the rainbow in your diet and this soup is the perfect starting point.

SPICY TOMATO AND RED PEPPER

Serves 4–6

4 tbsp rapeseed oil

2 large onions, chopped

3 garlic cloves, chopped

1 small carrot, chopped

4 red peppers, seeded and diced

1½ tsp chilli paste

400 g (14 oz) canned chopped tomatoes

1 litre (1¾ pints) vegetable stock

Salt, and freshly ground black pepper

Chilli flakes or sauce (optional)

Caramelise the onion in the oil (see *page 34*).

Add the garlic, carrot, red peppers and chilli paste. Cook on a medium to low heat, stirring well, until the vegetables become tender.

Add the chopped tomatoes followed by the vegetable stock. Bring everything to the boil, then turn down the heat and simmer, partially covered, until the carrot pieces are soft.

Take off the heat and blend the soup until smooth. Season to taste and add a few chilli flakes or some chilli sauce, if you like.

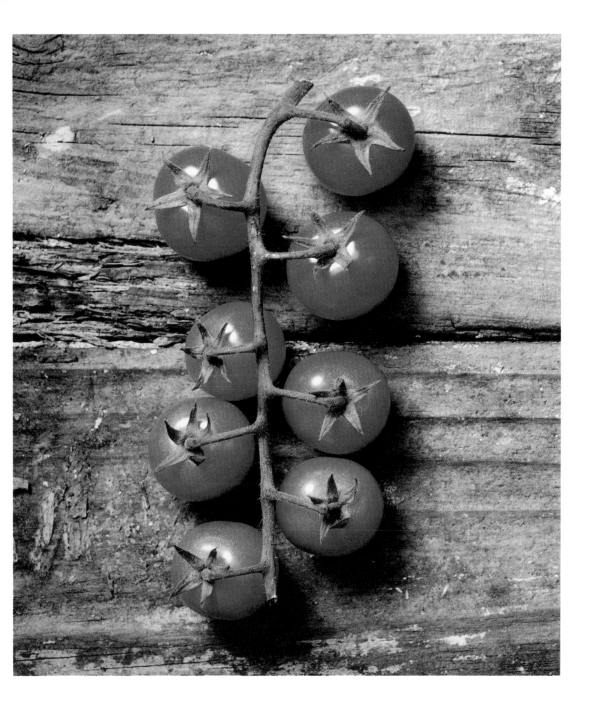

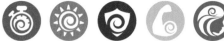

This is one of the very first soups I made and sold, and the reaction I received at the market stall was so positive that I credit this soup with convincing me to go ahead with my idea for a healthy soup company. The lentils add extra fibre to this rich tomato soup and give it a lovely velvety texture. Cooked tomatoes are rich in lycopene, a really powerful antioxidant that helps to keep cell membranes healthy. With the high vegetable content and a really good blend, there's just no reason to add any cream to this soup.

TOMATO AND RED LENTIL SOUP

Serves 4

2 tbsp rapeseed oil

I large onion, chopped

2 small garlic cloves, chopped

I medium carrot, chopped

5 celery sticks, chopped

I bay leaf

90 g (3¼ oz) dried red split lentils

400 g (14 oz) canned chopped tomatoes

750 ml (1¼ pints) vegetable stock

Salt and freshly ground black pepper

Caramelise the onion in the oil until golden (see *page 34*). Add the garlic, carrot and celery. Stir, then add the bay leaf and cook on a medium heat, partially covered, for around 10 minutes, until the vegetables are tender. Stir regularly.

Put the lentils into a sieve and rinse with cold water, then allow to drain and add to the vegetables, stirring them in. Keep stirring for a couple of minutes, then add the tomatoes.

Stir well again, then pour in the hot vegetable stock and bring to the boil. Turn down the heat and simmer, partially covered, for about 20 minutes, until the lentils are soft. You'll need to keep stirring the soup regularly to make sure that the lentils do not stick to the base of the pan.

Remove the bay leaf carefully with a spoon and take off the heat. Blend the soup until it is completely smooth, then season to taste. Stir in the seasoning well or give the soup another quick blitz of the blender, and your soup is ready to serve.

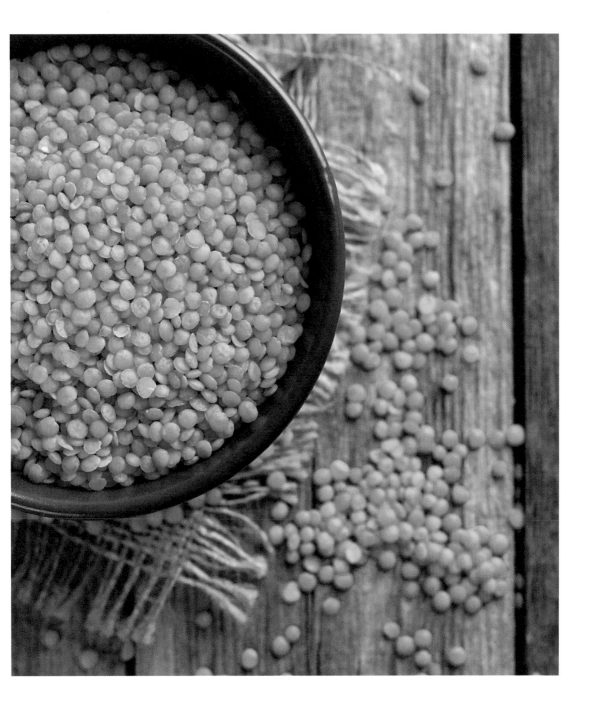

This refreshingly rich soup is best eaten chilled, but it is also delicious when warmed through. The aniseed taste of the fennel becomes mellow in the cooking and leaves a pleasing depth of flavour. This isn't a traditional gazpacho, which would normally have peppers and cucumber, but it's an interesting variation that's always very popular in my household – even among those who are not naturally fennel fans.

TOMATO AND FENNEL GAZPACHO

Serves 4–6

2 tbsp rapeseed oil

1 large onion, chopped

1 garlic clove, chopped

1 fennel bulb, trimmed and chopped

¼ tsp dried oregano

¾ tsp coriander seeds

⅓ tsp black peppercorns

200 g (7 oz) canned chopped tomatoes

2 tsp tomato purée

1.4 litres (2½ pints) vegetable stock

1 tsp agave nectar

Salt and freshly ground black pepper

Caramelise the onion in the oil (see *page 34*).

Add the garlic, fennel, oregano, coriander seeds and black peppercorns. Let the vegetables sweat on a medium to low heat, partially covered, for around 10 minutes, until the fennel is tender.

Add the chopped tomatoes and tomato purée and cook for another minute, stirring in well.

Add the vegetable stock, agave nectar, and salt and pepper, and bring to the boil. Then turn down the heat and simmer, partially covered, for around 5 minutes.

Take off the heat and blend until smooth, and season again, to taste, if needed. Leave the soup to cool, then cover and chill before serving. Decorate with the fennel fronds, if you like.

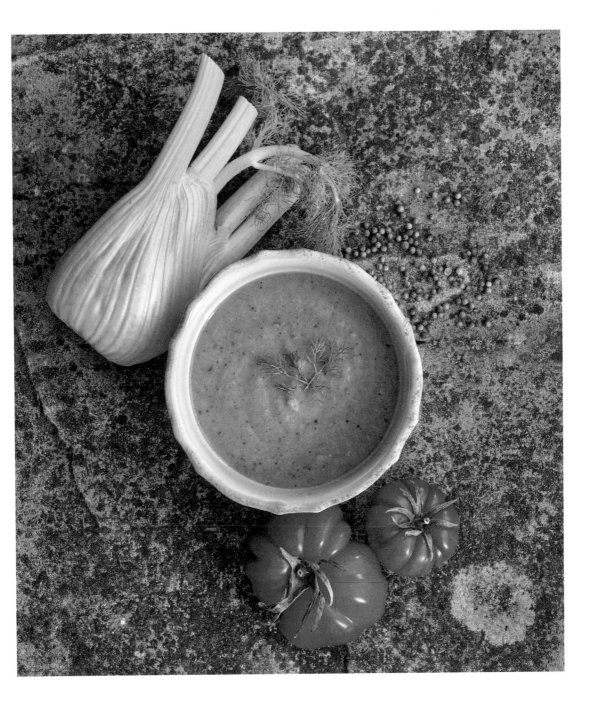

This is a characterful, chunky soup full of colour and verve, like a bright Mexican sombrero! The little green okra are really low in calories but are a rich source of fibre, minerals and vitamins. Be creative with toppings: cheese, salsa, chipotle flakes, a splash of extra lime or, of course, crunchy tortilla chips all work brilliantly well.

VEGAN TORTILLA SOUP

Serves 6

1½ tbsp rapeseed oil

2 medium onions, chopped

2 garlic cloves, peeled and chopped

1 red pepper, seeded and chopped

6 small okra, trimmed and chopped

130 g (4½ oz) sweetcorn (tinned or frozen)

½ red chilli, seeded and finely chopped (optional)

1 tbsp mild curry powder

400 g (14 oz) canned chopped tomatoes

1 tbsp chia seeds

1 litre (1¾ pints) vegetable stock

400 g (14 oz) canned black beans

1 tbsp fresh lime juice

Salt and freshly ground black pepper

Several sprigs of fresh coriander or parsley

Tortilla chips (optional)

Grated Cheddar cheese (optional)

Caramelise the onion in the oil (*see page 34*). Add the garlic, red pepper, okra, sweetcorn, chilli (if using) and curry powder. Cook on a gentle heat for 5 minutes, stirring frequently.

Add the chopped tomatoes, chia seeds and vegetable stock and mix in well. Simmer gently for approximately 20 minutes until all the vegetables are tender.

Wash and drain the beans, add them to the vegetables, and continue to simmer for a further 5 minutes.

Take off the heat, add the lime juice, season to taste, and then serve with a sprinkling of coriander (or parsley), and top with grated cheese if desired, and tortilla chips (a must in our household!).

Souper Tip Recipes often tell you to add ground spices towards the end of the cooking process. However, I find that adding them at the start, along with the vegetables, helps them to release their oils, thereby enhancing the flavour of the soup. It also prevents that gritty, granular texture that sometimes occurs when the spices are added too late in the cooking process.

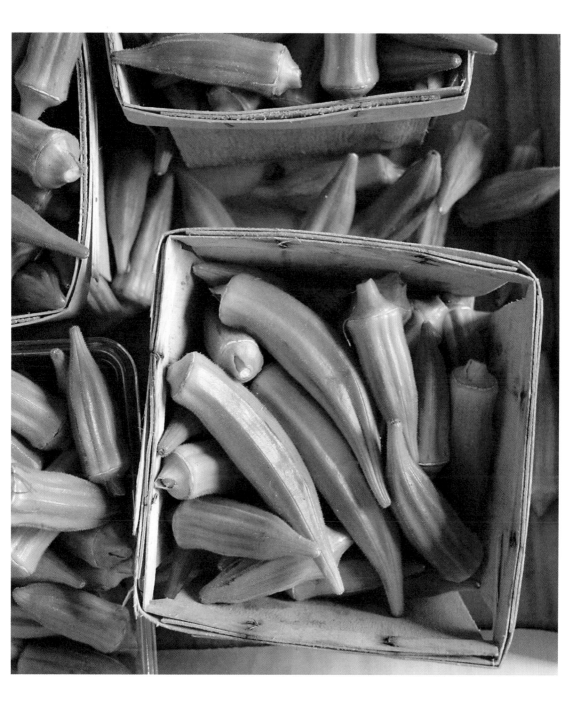

This is one of my 'swavoury' soups, as an American friend once said (see *page 15*). I admit that it does have a few surprises in the ingredients list, but I love this combination! The cucumber and strawberries make it a wonderfully hydrating soup, which is fruity and refreshing without being sickly sweet. It's a real winner for long, warm summer evenings. It is also incredibly quick and easy to make, which is just what you need for days when a hot kitchen is the last place you want to be. Keep back a few sprigs of tarragon for a pretty topping, if you like.

RAW STRAWBERRY AND TARRAGON

Serves 4

400 g (14 oz) hulled strawberries
¼ small red onion, roughly chopped
½ red pepper, roughly chopped
¼ cucumber, roughly chopped
¼ garlic clove
2 sprigs fresh tarragon
2 tsp balsamic vinegar
1½ tbsp olive oil
Pinch of pink Himalayan rock salt
Pinch of ground black pepper

Put everything into a blender (or food processor).

Blend until really smooth.

Pour into a bowl and chill. This soup is best served really cold.

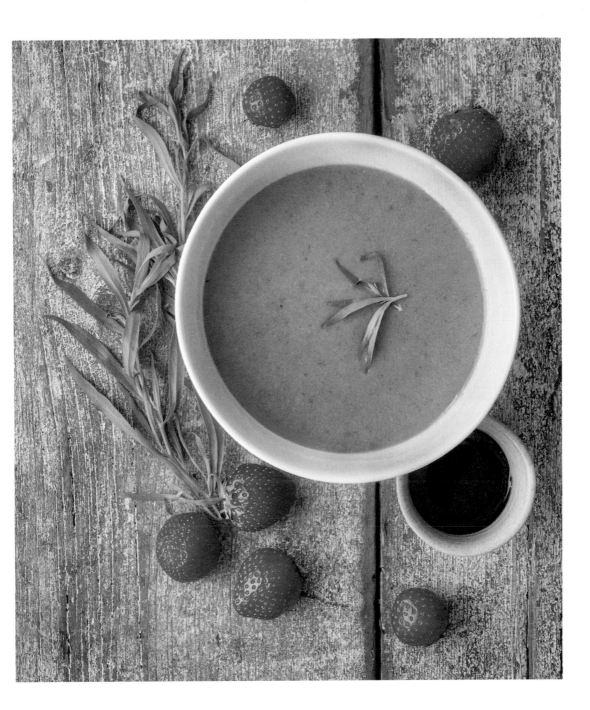

Move over Wimbledon! This revitalising soup will remind you that there is more to strawberries than dousing them in cream. I love strawberries, and here – with the sharp balsamic and a hint of heat from the ginger providing beautiful contrasts to the fruit – I've created a soup that really is a champion. High in vitamin C, strawberries are beneficial to the immune system. It seems criminal to save them for an event that only happens once a year!

STRAWBERRY WITH MELON SOUP

Serves 6

1 small cantaloupe melon

1 tbsp maple syrup

1 tbsp water

300 g (10 oz) fresh, hulled strawberries

½ tsp balsamic vinegar

1 cm (½ in) piece fresh root ginger, peeled and grated

Agave nectar (optional)

Put everything together into a blender (or food processor) and blend until smooth.

If desired, add agave nectar to sweeten further. Chill for a couple of hours before serving.

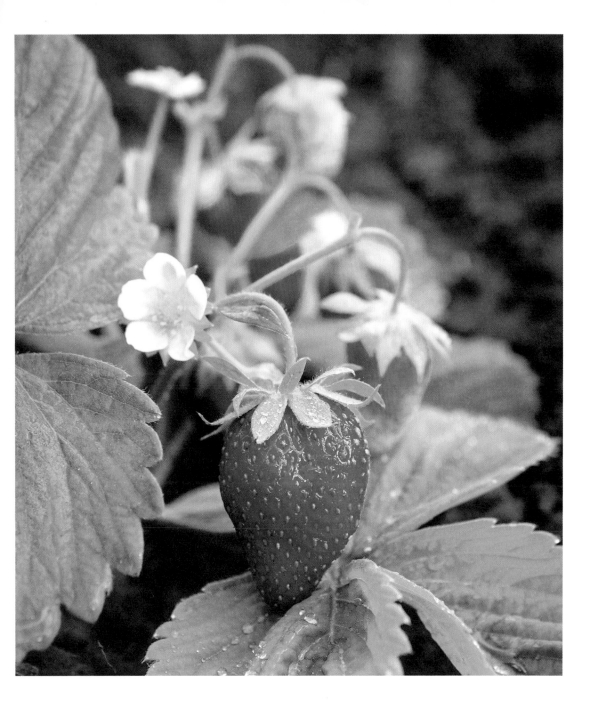

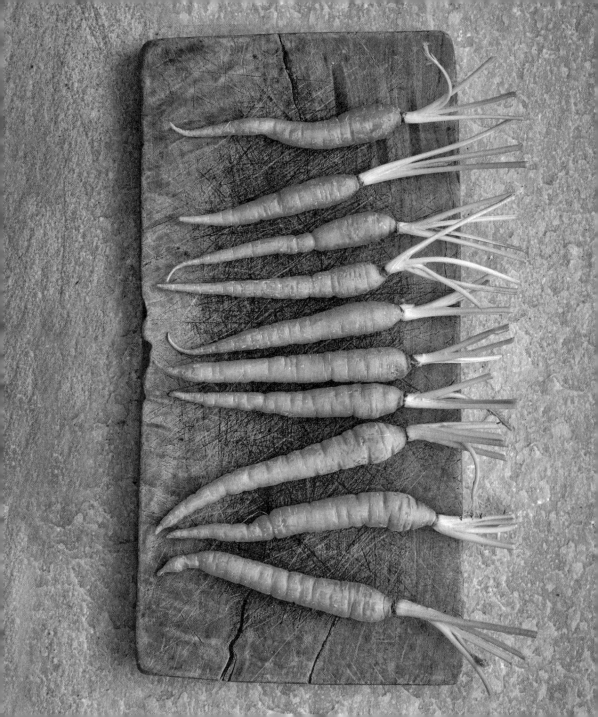

THE ORANGE SOUPS

Vibrant orange can do more than just lift your spirits. You probably know that orange fruit and veg are great for immunity due to their high Vitamin C content, but did you know that betacarotene, found in sweet potatoes, apricot and carrots, can also contribute to a healthy immune system? The deeper the orange, the greater the goodness – and you will be able to see the benefits, as orange veggies also have your vision covered. The Butternut Squash and Sweet Potato is a comforting autumnal favourite while Mango and Coconut guarantees to transport you to warmer days.

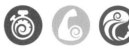

The butterbean seems a bit old-fashioned these days, what with the rise in profile of beans like cannellini, pinto, black-eyed and adzuki. But I love using butterbeans in soups, because I find that the distinctive creamy flavour and buttery texture makes them exceptionally smooth and comforting. These beans are a really well-rounded source of nutrition too, providing fibre, protein, iron, carbs and B vitamins. They're a low-energy-density food, meaning that compared to the size of the serving, they are really low in calories, so you can eat lots of them and feel really full, but without worrying about putting on weight. In this soup, where I've also included carrots and some lovely herbs and spices, you'll be reminded of just how good these familiar beans can taste. Top with a little fresh parsley, if you like.

BUTTERBEAN AND CARROT

Serves 4

1 tbsp rapeseed oil
1 small onion, peeled and diced
1 garlic clove, peeled and chopped
2 large carrots, peeled and diced
1 large potato, peeled and diced
1 tsp mustard seed
200 g (7 oz) canned butterbeans
Pinch cayenne pepper
630 ml (21 fl oz) vegetable stock
1 tsp dried parsley
Pinch of salt

Caramelise the onion in the oil (see *page 34*).

Add the garlic, carrot and potato, and cook for around 20 minutes, partially covered, on a medium to low heat until the vegetables become tender.

Drain the butterbeans (there is no need to wash). Add the mustard seeds and stir in well before adding the butterbeans and cayenne pepper.

Add the vegetable stock and bring to the boil, then turn down the heat and simmer, partially covered, for around 5 minutes, until the vegetables are soft.

Add the dried parsley and salt, and cook for a further minute. This is a chunky soup, so no blending is required.

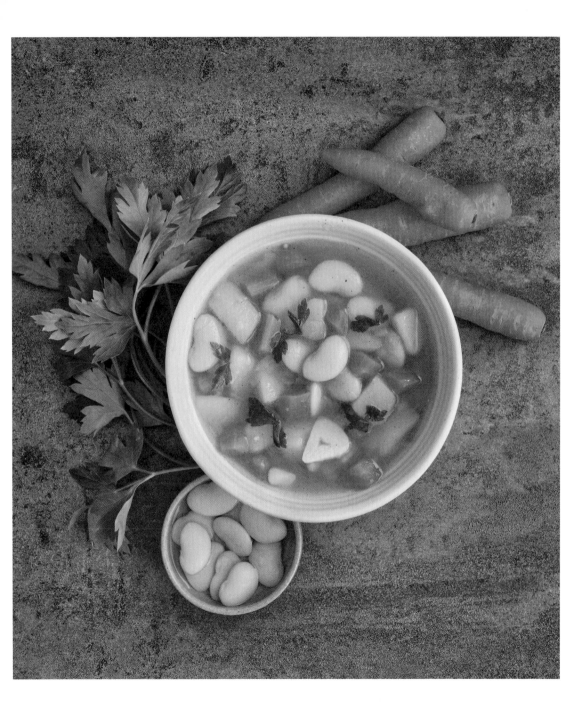

This soup is perfect for those times when you find yourself hankering after some healthy, hearty flavours to keep you warm and full. Butternut squash and sweet potato complement each other really well, and I feel more cheerful just seeing their bright colours in a bowl. This combination also makes a wonderfully creamy and rich pasta sauce and goes perfectly with risotto. It's also a soup that I always keep handy in the freezer, in case of unexpected guests or emergencies.

BUTTERNUT SQUASH AND SWEET POTATO

Serves 5–6

2 tbsp rapeseed oil

1 large onion, chopped

1 leek, trimmed and chopped

½ butternut squash (about 650 g/23 oz), peeled and diced

2 medium sweet potatoes, peeled and diced

Generous pinch ground nutmeg

¼ tsp ground ginger

1 litre (1¾ pints) vegetable stock

100 g (3½ oz) coconut cream

Salt and freshly ground black pepper

Caramelise the onion in the oil (*see page 34*). Add the leek, butternut squash and sweet potato and let the vegetables sweat for 5–6 minutes, partially covered. Stir occasionally.

Add the nutmeg and ginger, mix in well, then add the vegetable stock. Stir well and bring to the boil. Then turn down the heat and simmer gently, partially covered, for around 10–15 minutes, until the butternut squash is completely cooked. Stir regularly.

Add the coconut cream and mix in well.

Take off the heat and blend the soup until completely smooth. Season to taste.

Souper Topper Some crunchy toasted coconut flakes sprinkled over the top make a pretty and nutritious addition to this soup. To toast the coconut: preheat the oven to 150°C/300°F/Gas Mark 2. Spread the coconut flakes on a dry baking sheet and bake in the oven for a few minutes. Keep watching and moving them around so they toast evenly to a light golden brown.

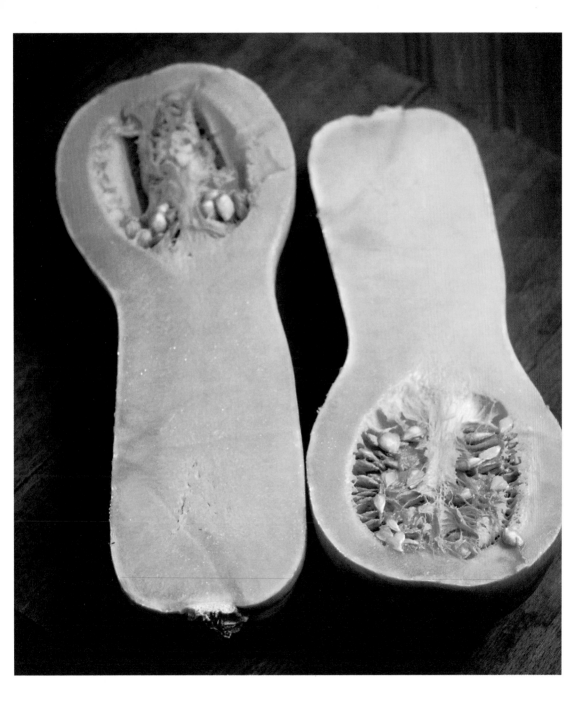

This was among our first soups and it still brings me such pleasure to lay out the vegetables on the baking tray, sprinkle them with nutmeg and oil and then wait, with delicious anticipation, for those roasting aromas to start wafting out of the oven. The red pepper and dash of lime gives the soup colour and zing, and nutritionally, this soup meets autumn's needs: just at the point we're all coming down with colds and coughs, this gives you a welcome shot of vitamins C and A, along with lots of betacarotene, to help fight off those pesky germs and viruses.

ROASTED BUTTERNUT AND RED PEPPER

Serves 4–6

½ large butternut squash, peeled, seeded and roughly chopped

1 red pepper, deseeded and roughly chopped

½ tsp ground nutmeg

2 tbsp rapeseed oil

1 large onion, chopped

1 garlic clove, peeled and chopped

850 ml (1½ pints) vegetable stock

1½ tsp fresh lime juice

Salt and freshly ground black pepper

Preheat the oven to 190°C/375°F/Gas mark 5. Arrange the squash and red pepper in a roasting tin, sprinkle over the nutmeg and mix well. Roast in the oven for around 30 minutes, until flecks of brown start to appear on the pepper pieces.

While you're waiting for the squash and peppers to roast, caramelise the onion in the oil (see page 34), then add the garlic and continue to cook, partially covered, for another couple of minutes.

Add the vegetable stock, stir and bring to the boil. Turn down the heat and simmer gently, partially covered, for 5 minutes.

Once the squash and pepper pieces are done, add them to the pan and stir well. Bring back to the boil then simmer gently, partially covered, for a few minutes.

Take off the heat, stir in the lime juice and blend until completely smooth. Season to taste. Popcorn is delicious as a topping on this soup.

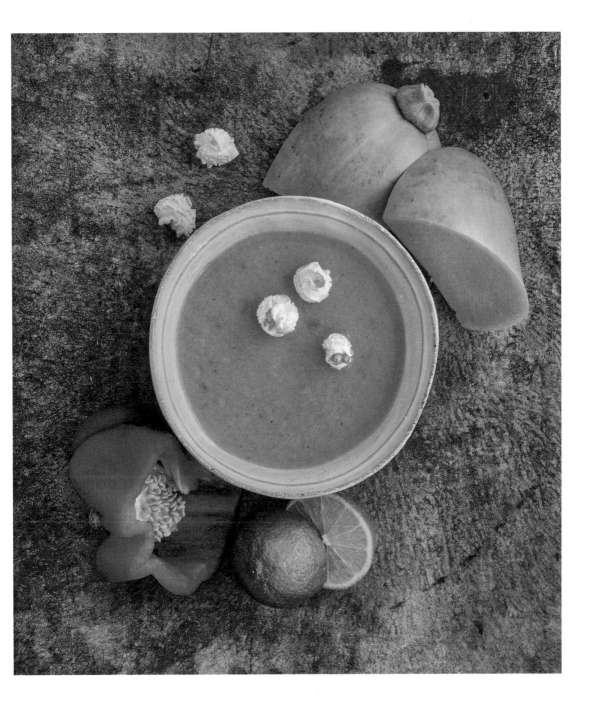

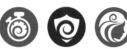

This Caribbean-inspired soup has a creamy and zesty flavour, with the coconut providing a more delicate flavour than traditional dairy cream. The lime juice helps all the flavours to sing and the spices create an exotic touch. It's good for you too, with the betacarotene in the carrots promoting healthy eyesight, while coconuts are rich in fibre and provide multiple vitamins. I like to have this soup gently warmed through, rather than boiling hot, as I find I can taste all the wonderful flavours much more vividly that way.

CREAMY CARROT WITH COCONUT AND LIME

Serves 4–5

2 tbsp rapeseed oil

1 large onion, chopped

1 tsp chilli paste

½ tsp ground turmeric

½ tsp ground coriander seeds

2 garlic cloves, peeled and chopped

1.25 cm (½ in) piece fresh root ginger, peeled and finely grated

1 large potato, peeled and chopped

3 medium carrots, peeled and chopped

350 ml (12 fl oz) vegetable stock

400 ml (14 fl oz) coconut milk

3 tsp fresh lime juice

Salt and freshly ground black pepper

Caramelise the onion in the oil (see page 34), then add the chilli paste, turmeric and coriander seeds and cook on a medium to low heat for about 1 minute.

Add the garlic and ginger and cook for a further minute.

Add the potatoes and carrots and let them sweat for 5–6 minutes, partially covered. Stir occasionally.

Add the vegetable stock, stir well and bring to the boil. Then turn down the heat and simmer gently, partially covered, for around 10 minutes, until the carrots are soft. Stir from time to time while cooking.

Turn up the heat, add the coconut milk and lime juice and stir in well. Then take off the heat and blend the soup until completely smooth. Season to taste.

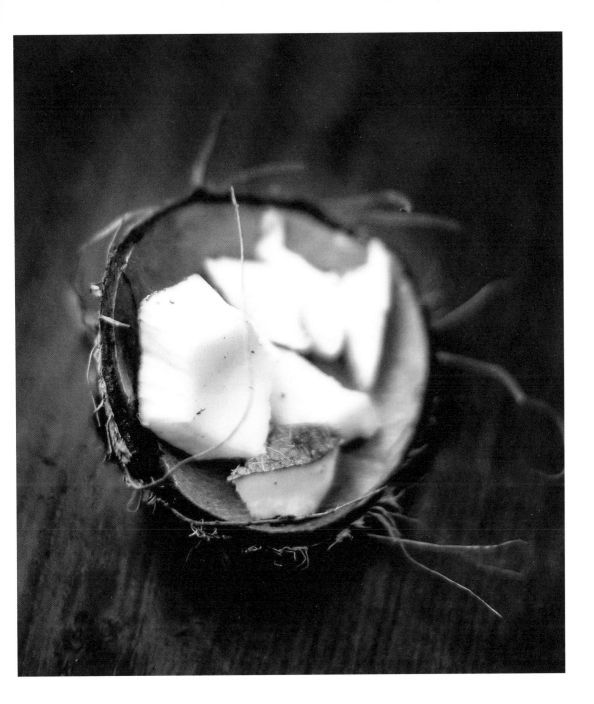

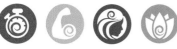

I find that Thai dishes contain a particularly fragrant blend of ingredients, which helps to give this cuisine its refreshing taste. This soup is a nod to that tradition, containing peanuts, coconut oil and chilli sauce, all of which combine to create a taste that really boosts the background carrot. Feel free to increase the chilli depending on your taste, but be careful not to over-season with salt, because the peanut butter adds a lot of salt of its own. Try sprinkling some chopped peanuts over the soup when you serve it, to add that extra crunch and texture. Benefits-wise, coconut oil is known as being particularly helpful to maintaining healthy hair and skin, as well as having antioxidant properties that promote good overall health. The peanuts, of course, pack a great protein punch.

THAI CARROT AND PEANUT

Serves 4–5

2 tbsp coconut oil

1 medium onion, chopped

3 garlic cloves, peeled and chopped

1 tsp chilli paste

650 g (1 lb 7 oz) carrots, peeled and chopped

1 litre (1¾ pints) vegetable stock

75 g (2½ oz) peanut butter

Pinch of salt

Agave nectar (optional)

Caramelise the onion in the coconut oil (see *page 34*).

Add the garlic, chilli paste and carrots to the onion and let the vegetables sweat for 5–6 minutes, partially covered. Stir occasionally.

Add the vegetable stock, stir well and bring to the boil. Turn down the heat and simmer gently, stirring occasionally, for around 10 minutes, until the carrots are soft.

Add the peanut butter and mix in well.

Take off the heat and blend the soup until completely smooth. Season to taste with salt (go easy!) and add a teaspoon of agave nectar, if you like.

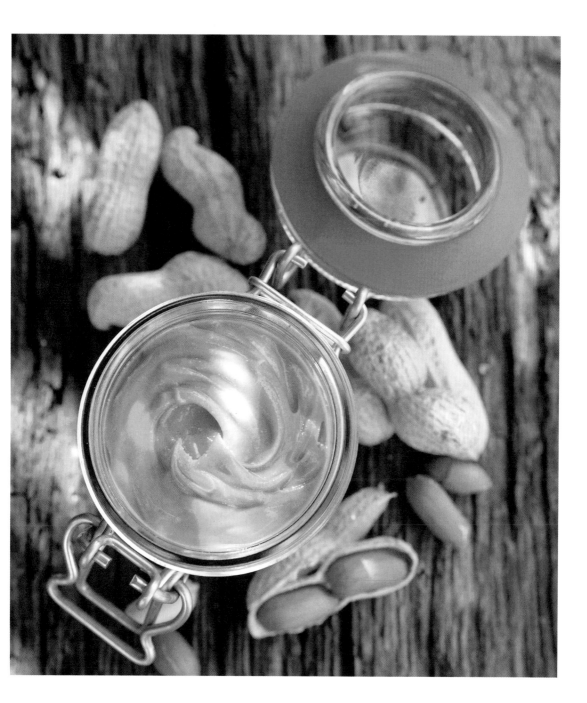

This is such a staple soup – you see it all the time in the supermarkets, along with its even more common cousin, Carrot and Coriander. It's so ubiquitous that virtually every soup company, fresh, canned and pasteurized, offers some version of it in their range. But if you look at the list of ingredients on the back of the packaging, it's obvious that it has usually been so messed around with that the taste is unrecognisable. Certainly it rarely tastes like the incredibly nourishing dish that it should be, bursting with betacarotene and vitamins A and C. So here's my very simple recipe, which strips back the cooking time and the ingredients to the bare minimum, allowing the taste of the carrots and herbs to come to the fore and bask in their own glory. The only thing I ask is that you buy the best quality carrots you can afford, because with such a simple recipe, the flavour of this soup will depend on the quality of your initial ingredients.

CARROT AND TARRAGON

Serves 4–6

3 tbsp rapeseed oil

1 large onion, chopped

5 carrots, peeled and chopped

2 leeks, chopped

1 litre (1¾ pints) vegetable stock

Pinch dried tarragon

2 tsp agave nectar

Salt and freshly ground black pepper

Caramelise the onion (*see page 34*).

Add the carrots and leeks to the onion and mix in well.

Cook on a medium to low heat, partially covered, for around 10 minutes, until the vegetables are tender. Stir occasionally.

Add the hot vegetable stock and bring to the boil. Then lower the heat and simmer, partially covered, for another 5 minutes or so, until the vegetables are cooked.

Add the tarragon and agave nectar, mix in well and continue to simmer for a further minute. Take off the heat, blend until completely smooth and season to taste.

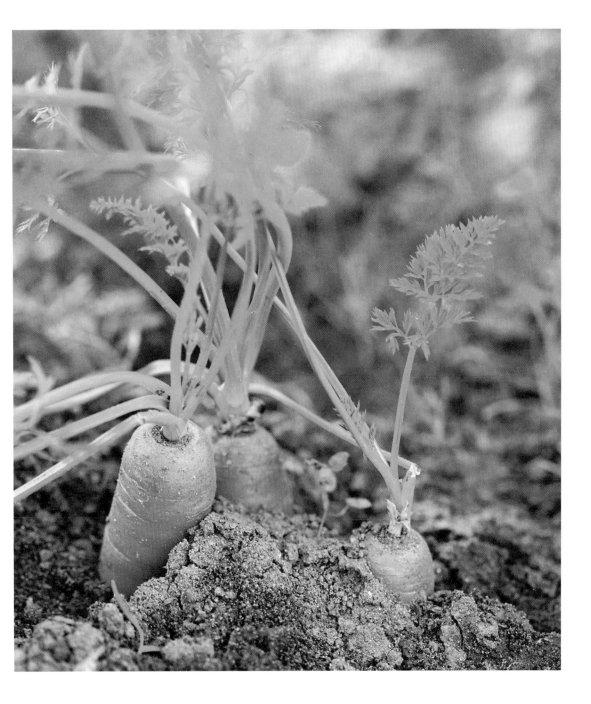

Middle Eastern dishes are very popular at the moment, from the humble hummus to the rich tomato goodness of shakshuka. All of us at Soupologie love the flavour-packed tastes of the Middle East, and za'atar is a spice combination that typifies this cuisine. Za'atar can consist of various spices, but I like the combination that contains toasted sesame seeds, oregano, thyme, coriander, marjoram, sumac, salt and cumin. This is a hybrid 'East meets West' soup, combining the sweet British carrot with the rich flavour of this ancient spice. Many of the spices in za'atar have anti-inflammatory and immune-boosting properties.

ROASTED CARROT WITH ZA'ATAR

Serves 5–6

For the roasted carrots

2 tbsp rapeseed oil

450 g (1 lb) carrots, peeled and chopped

2 garlic cloves, whole and unpeeled

2 tbsp za'atar

For the remainder of the soup

1 tsp turmeric

3 tbsp tomato purée

400 g (14 oz) canned cannellini beans

1.25 litres (2 pints) vegetable stock

2 tsp fresh lemon juice

Salt and freshly ground black pepper

Preheat the oven to 190°C/375°F/Gas mark 5. Begin by roasting the carrots. Line a roasting tin with baking parchment and put the carrots, garlic and za'atar into the tin, pour over the oil and mix together well. Roast for 30–35 minutes.

Remove the tin from the oven and, being careful not to touch the sides, pick out the garlic cloves and squeeze out the cooked flesh, discarding the skins.

Wash and drain the beans. Using the baking parchment, transfer the entire contents of the roasting tin to a separate pan. Add the turmeric, tomato purée and beans and cook on a medium heat for 3–4 minutes. Pour in the vegetable stock, stir well and bring to the boil.

Turn down the heat and simmer gently for 4–5 minutes, stirring occasionally. Add the lemon juice and mix well. Take off the heat and blend the soup until completely smooth. Season to taste and sprinkle with toasted sesame seeds, if you like.

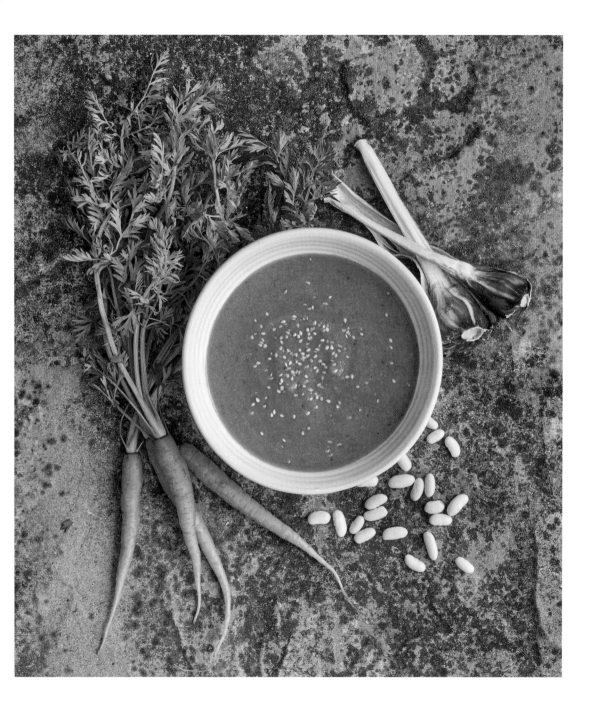

This is the soup I make for family and friends when I hear the first sneeze of the season. I usually make a large batch and freeze most of it, so I can always whip some out and serve it up to the patient as quickly as possible. Apart from all the vitamins and nutrients that come from the carrots, added Vitamin C appears via the orange, and that hit of ginger is just enough to soothe a sore throat and clear the nose. It's an easy set of ingredients to have to hand and a soup that will never let you down in terms of delivering some souper nourishment, just when you need it.

CARROT, ORANGE AND GINGER

Serves 3–4

2 tbsp rapeseed oil

1 large onion, chopped

1 garlic clove, peeled and chopped

6 medium carrots, peeled and chopped

1 tsp grated orange zest

1.25 cm (½ in) piece fresh root ginger, peeled and finely grated

200 g (7 oz) canned chopped tomatoes

750 ml (1¼ pints) vegetable stock

1 tbsp orange juice

1 tsp agave nectar (optional)

Salt and freshly ground black pepper

Caramelise the onion in the oil (see page 34), then add the garlic, carrot, orange zest and ginger. (Keep back a little orange zest for topping, if you like.)

Allow the vegetables to sweat for 5–6 minutes, partially covered. Stir occasionally.

Add the tomatoes and vegetable stock to the vegetable mixture, stir, and bring to the boil. Then turn down the heat and simmer gently, partially covered, for around 10 minutes, until the carrots are soft.

Add the orange juice and agave nectar (if you want to add more sweetness) and stir in well.

Take off the heat and blend the soup until completely smooth. Season to taste and sprinkle with a little orange zest to add an attractive finishing touch.

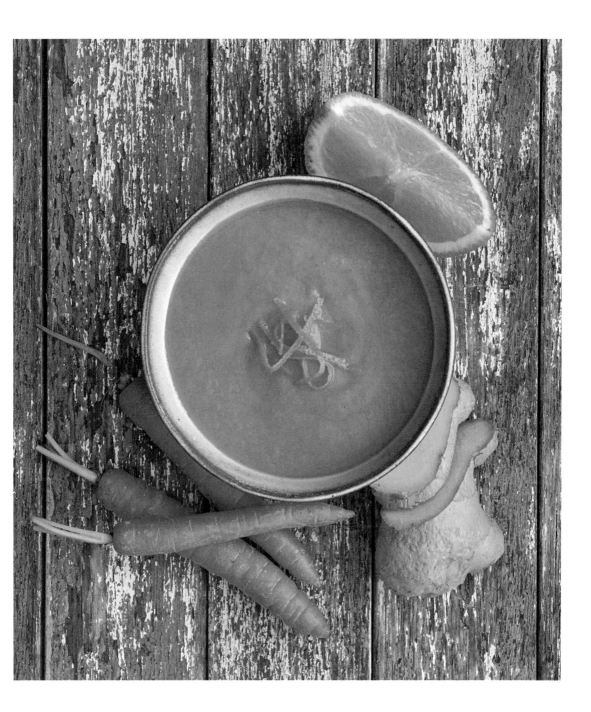

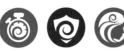

This is a thick creamy soup with spices that will warm you up and make you glow from the inside out. As you make your way through the bowl, the spicy notes seem to mellow and end up leaving you with a gentle heat at the back of the mouth. If you prefer something more fiery, use a stronger curry powder, but this milder version should suit most people and it allows the taste of the vegetables to keep to the forefront. Full of amazing nutrients, these two vegetables blend together so well, you'll keep coming back for more.

CURRIED PARSNIP AND SWEET POTATO

Serves 4–5

2 tbsp rapeseed oil

1 large onion, chopped

1 garlic clove, peeled and chopped

4 medium parsnips, peeled and chopped

1 small sweet potato, peeled and chopped

20 g (¾ oz) mild curry powder

750 ml (1¼ pints) vegetable stock

65 ml (2¼ fl oz) creamed coconut

Salt and freshly ground black pepper

Caramelise the onion in the oil (see *page 34*).

Add the garlic, parsnip, sweet potato and curry powder to the onions. Let the vegetables sweat for 5–6 minutes, partially covered. Stir occasionally.

Add the vegetable stock, stir and bring to the boil. Then turn down the heat and simmer gently, partially covered, for around 15 minutes, until the parsnips are soft. Stir occasionally.

Add the creamed coconut and stir in well. Take off the heat and blend the soup until completely smooth. Season to taste.

Souper Tip This soup is delicious with a sprinkling of toasted coconut flakes. To toast the flakes, spread them on a dry baking sheet and bake in the oven on a low setting (150°C/300°F/Gas Mark 2) for a few minutes. Keep watching and moving them around so they are toasted evenly and turn golden brown.

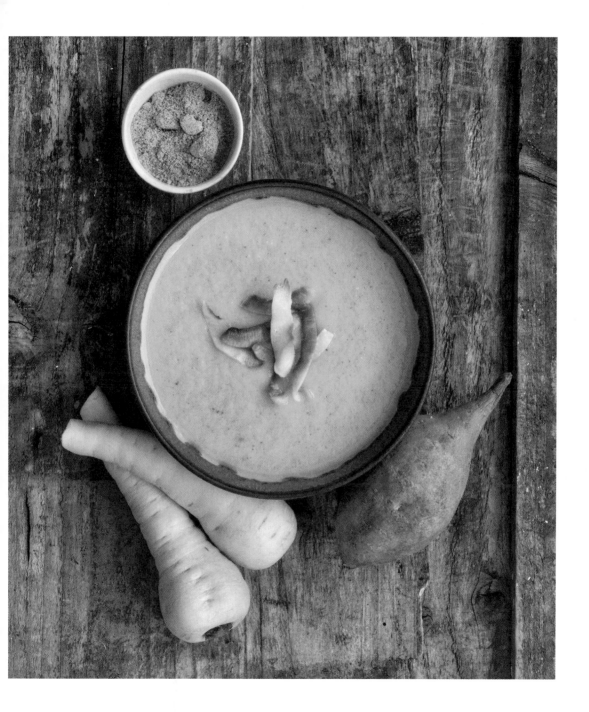

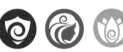

This soup provides a wonderful harmony of contrasting flavours. It is deliciously sweet, thanks mainly to the roasted sweet potato, which is complemented beautifully by the Middle-Eastern-inspired 'pesto'. Healthwise, this soup is packed with vitamins and the pistachios are both a source of fibre and full of 'good fats' that help to give you a lasting full feeling. The mint works to aid digestion as well as providing an important flavour balance to this recipe.

SWEET POTATO SOUP WITH PISTACHIO, ORANGE AND MINT PESTO

Serves 4–5

For the soup

3 tbsp rapeseed oil

I small onion, peeled and chopped

3 garlic cloves, peeled and chopped

2 carrots, peeled and chopped

4 sweet potatoes, peeled and chopped

4 sage leaves, finely chopped

I litre (1¾ pints) vegetable stock

¼ tsp nutmeg

30 ml (1 fl oz) fresh orange juice

For the pesto

I tbsp grated orange zest

45 g (1½ oz) shelled pistachio nuts

I spring onion, trimmed and sliced

I tbsp mint leaves

½ tsp salt

75 ml (2½ fl oz) olive oil

Caramelise the onion in the oil (*see page 34*).

Add the garlic, carrot, sweet potato and sage leaves. Let the vegetables sweat for 5–6 minutes, partially covered. Stir regularly.

Add the vegetable stock and nutmeg, stir and bring to the boil. Then turn down the heat and simmer gently, partially covered, for around 15 minutes, until the carrot and sweet potato pieces are soft. Stir occasionally.

While the vegetables are simmering, put all the ingredients for the pesto into a separate bowl and blend until completely emulsified, then set aside.

Once the soup is ready, take off the heat, add the orange juice, and blend the soup until completely smooth. Season to taste.

Serve by pouring the soup into a bowl and swirling some of the pesto into the centre.

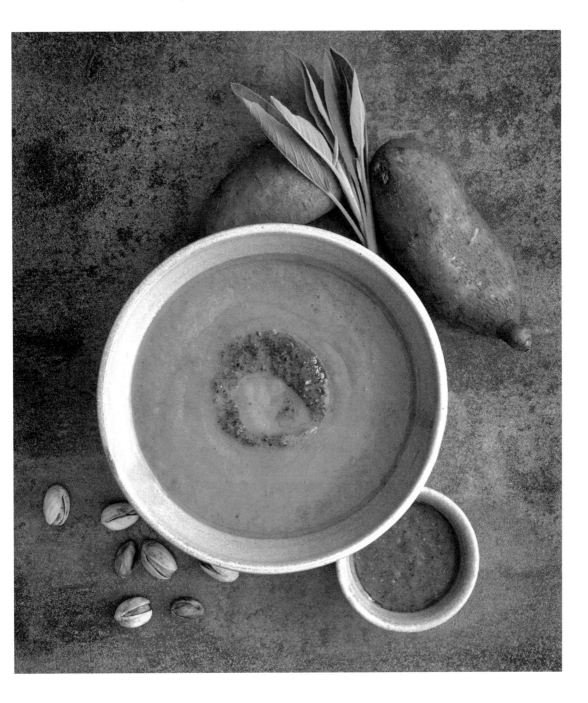

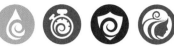

The flavour and aroma of apricots are like an instant holiday – they transport me straight to a hot climate, perhaps on a sun lounger next to a glistening pool. But back to reality – this soup is great in the winter, when fresh fruit is more expensive, and the vivid colour is like a ray of sunshine in your bowl. Did you know that dried apricots actually contain more potassium and fibre per 100 g (3½ oz) than their fresh counterparts? As if you didn't have enough reasons to get cooking! This soup can be enjoyed warmed or chilled.

APRICOT SOUP

Serves 6

250 g (9 oz) dried apricots
1 tbsp fresh lemon juice
1 tsp grated lemon zest
½ tbsp cornflour
Agave nectar (optional)

Place the apricots in a bowl and add 250 ml (8½ fl oz) of boiling water. Leave for half an hour or so, until the apricots are rehydrated.

Transfer the apricots and their soaking water into a pan. Add 750 ml (1¼ pints) of water and bring to the boil.

Turn down the heat and simmer, partially covered, for 20–30 minutes until the apricots are completely soft.

Add the lemon juice and zest to the pan.

In a cup, mix the cornflour with a small amount of cold water to make a smooth paste. Turn the heat beneath the saucepan to low, and stir the cornflour paste into the soup. Continue to stir constantly while bringing it back to the boil – the mixture will thicken as it reaches boiling point.

Take the soup off the heat and blend. Add 1 tbsp of agave nectar if you wish to sweeten the soup slightly and blend again.

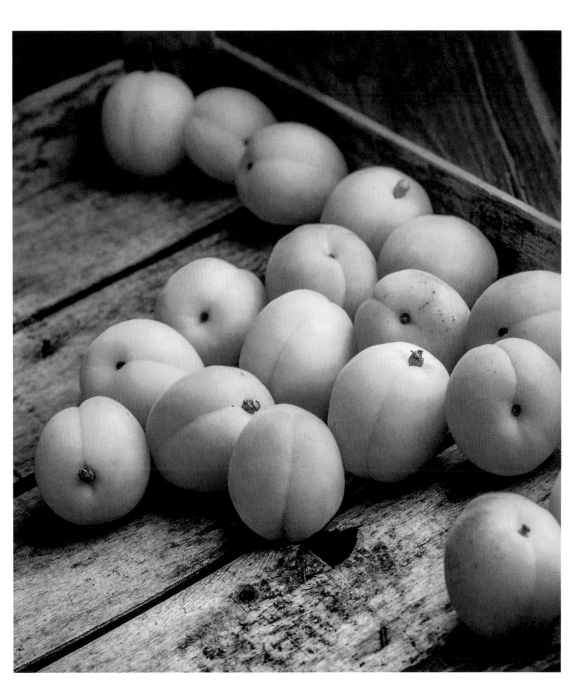

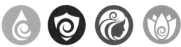

Quick and easy, this soup is perfect for when you need a nutritional boost and fast! Often overlooked, cantaloupe melon is in fact packed with vitamins and minerals – gram for gram, it has 30 times the betacarotene content of oranges. And I am sure you can guess what's coming: full of fibre and water, it is also a very low-energy-density food! The little tipple of wine in this soup gives it a perfect kick, and it pairs brilliantly with the sweet mango to make a deliciously refreshing meal. Making this soup could not be easier.

MANGO, MELON AND COCONUT SOUP

Serves 6

2 mangos, peeled, stoned and chopped

350 g (12 oz) cantaloupe melon, peeled, seeded and chopped

1 tbsp fresh lemon juice

75 ml (2½ fl oz) dry white wine

2 tbsp coconut yoghurt

Put all the ingredients into a blender and blend until completely smooth.

Place into a bowl and chill.

Serve cold, topped with toasted coconut flakes (*see page 112*) or fresh mint leaves.

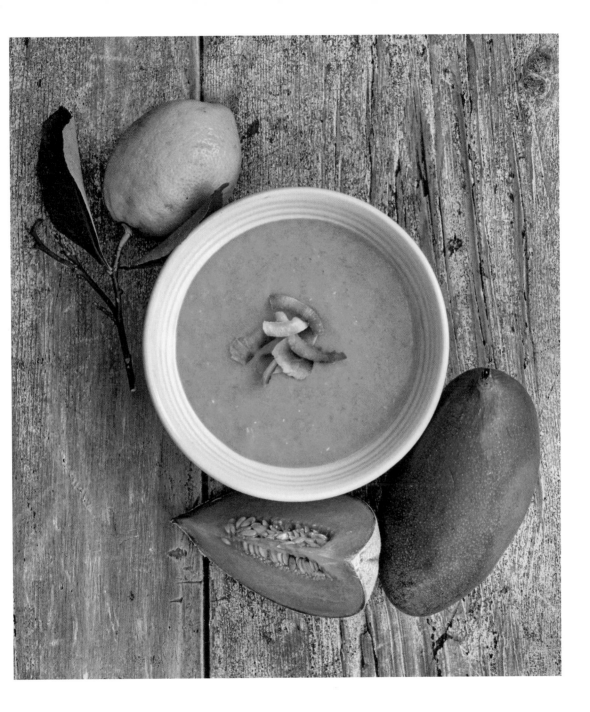

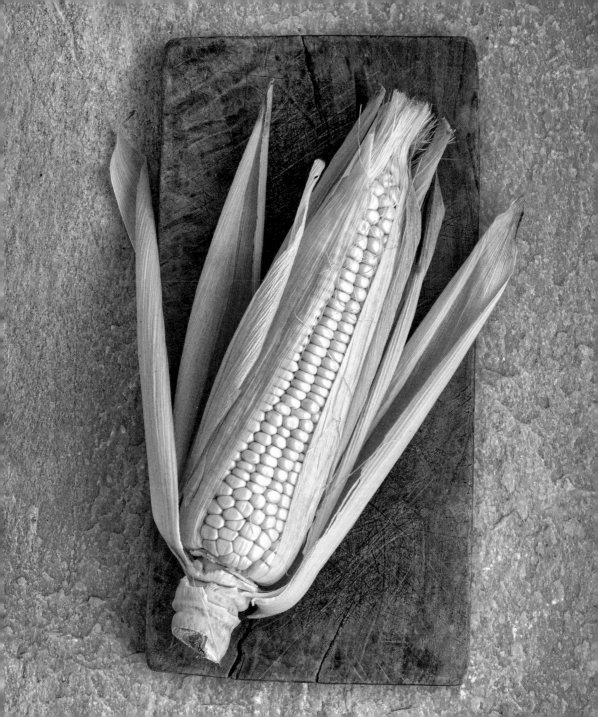

THE YELLOW SOUPS

We tend to associate yellow with sunshine and happiness, and for good reason! Turmeric is one of the most powerful super spices on the planet, while citrussy lime helps you get your Vitamin C hit. Comfort veg such as corn and potatoes also help to bring a boost of yellow to your soups, along with vitamins and minerals that are bound to keep a smile on your face.

My own twist on the familiar Leek and Potato or Vichysoisse soup is this 'golden' version which includes carrots for all sorts of extra benefits. Carrots can be traced back about 5,000 years, and in ancient times were grown for medicine, not food. They bring large amounts of Vitamin A and antioxidants to the party, which may help to keep blood sugar regulated and improve immune function. This recipe allows the sweetness of the carrots to beautifully complement the leeks and the milder potatoes, and you can enjoy the soup chilled as well as hot. If you feel like spicing it up a bit, feel free to add a potato-friendly spice or herb such as a mild curry powder, paprika or rosemary – but not all three at once!

GOLDEN LEEK AND POTATO

Serves 4

1½ tbsp rapeseed oil

1 small onion, peeled and diced

1 garlic clove, peeled and diced

1½ carrots, peeled and diced

3 medium leeks, washed, trimmed and diced

1 large potato, peeled and diced

¼ tsp nutmeg

½ tsp mustard powder

750 ml (1¼ pints) vegetable stock

Pinch dried oregano

Salt and freshly ground black pepper

Caramelise the onion in the oil for 4–5 minutes (see *page 34*).

Add the garlic, carrot, leek and potato. Cook on medium to low heat for around 15 minutes, until the vegetables are tender.

Add the nutmeg and mustard powder to the vegetables, followed by the stock. Bring to the boil, then lower the heat and simmer, partially covered, until the vegetables are cooked. This will take another 15 minutes or so.

Add the oregano and cook for a further minute. Take off the heat, blend until completely smooth and season to taste.

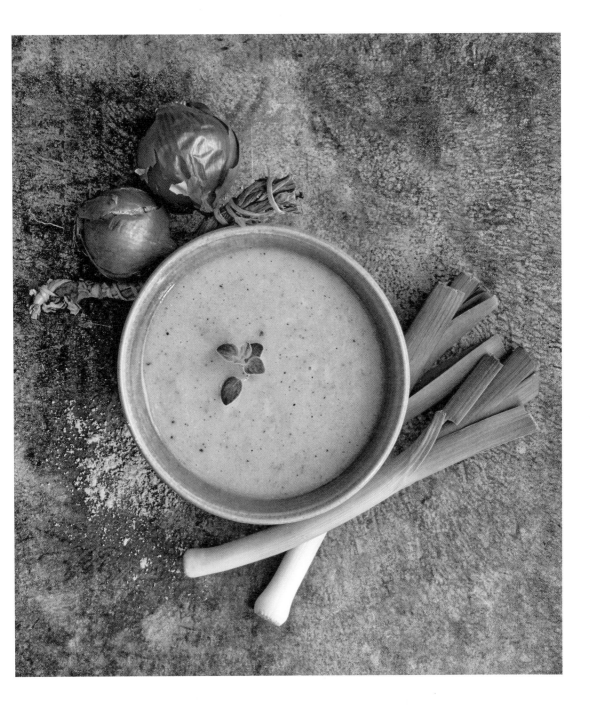

What a long way seaweed has come! There are a myriad of varieties that are easily available now, although I think that kombu works best in this soup. It's packed full of nutrients, including iodine, glutamic acid (associated with lower blood pressure), calcium, magnesium, potassium and iron. This recipe combines it with sweetcorn for a really thick creamy soup that is truly a meal in itself. You are unlikely to need any additional salt as the seaweed does the job of seasoning perfectly well. If you want to add texture and a little pizzazz, try floating some roasted sweetcorn *(see page 38)* and chopped chives on the top, or even plain popcorn (which works surprisingly well and packs a useful punch of magnesium).

CORN CHOWDER WITH SEAWEED

Serves 4

1 tbsp rapeseed oil

1 small onion, chopped

1 garlic clove, chopped

2 small potatoes, peeled and chopped

200 g (7 oz) frozen sweetcorn

½ tsp ground coriander

1 strip kombu seaweed

650 ml (22 fl oz) vegetable stock

Ground black pepper

Caramelise the onion in the oil *(see page 34)*.

Add the garlic, potatoes, sweetcorn, seaweed and coriander.

Sweat the vegetables for about 20 minutes, on a medium to low heat, until the potatoes become tender. Keep stirring so that none of the ingredients burn on the bottom of the pan.

Add the vegetable stock, bring to the boil, then reduce the heat and simmer, partially covered, for 8–10 minutes, until the vegetables are soft.

Take off the heat and blend the soup until smooth. Add pepper to taste, and serve sprinkled with roasted corn kernels, chopped chives or plain popcorn.

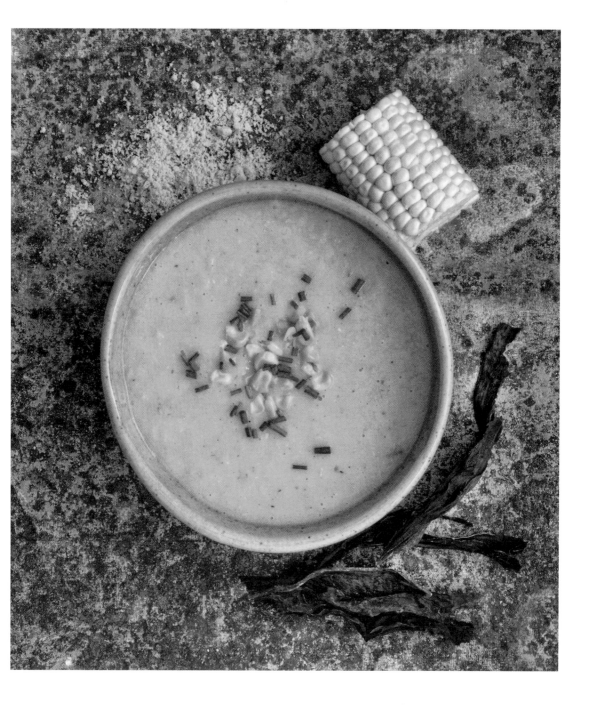

Lightly spiced, zingy and sweet, this fruit soup is a favourite at the Soupologie HQ. Ginger and cardamom are both known for being anti-inflammatory and helping to control cholesterol, so they are useful in lowering the risk of heart disease. The citrus juices add a burst of Vitamin C and antioxidants, as do the peaches, which contain phenolic compounds that have anti-obesity and anti-inflammatory effects. So you have the perfect excuse to treat yourself to this slightly exotic and utterly delicious fruit soup – drink away as your heart so rightly desires.

PEACH AND COCONUT SOUP

Serves 6

900 g (2 lb) fresh peaches, peeled, stoned and sliced

250 ml (8½ fl oz) fresh orange juice

250 ml (8½ fl oz) fresh peach juice

60 ml (2 fl oz) fresh lime juice

2 tbsp clear honey

I tsp ground ginger

½ tsp ground cardamom

½ tsp ground cinnamon

2 cloves

120 ml (4 fl oz) coconut yoghurt

In a large pan, combine everything except the yoghurt and bring the mixture to a boil.

Simmer, partially covered, for about 10 to 15 minutes or until the peaches are soft. Stir regularly while cooking.

Leave to cool, then remove and discard the cloves.

Pour the soup mixture into a blender and process until smooth.

Stir in the yoghurt and refrigerate for at least 4 hours before serving.

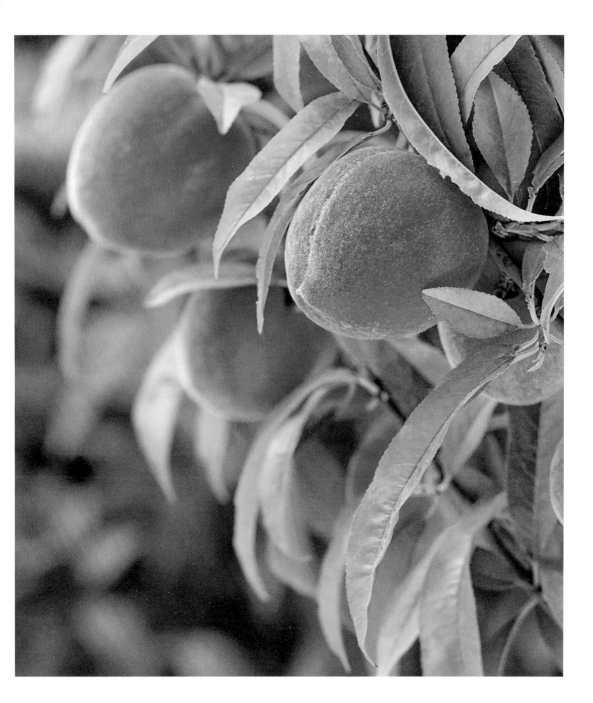

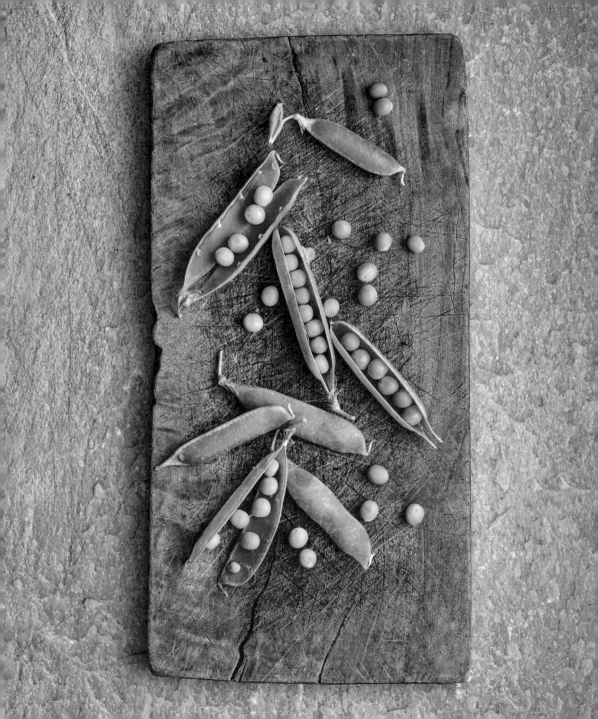

THE GREEN SOUPS

You probably don't need reminding why it's great to go green, but I am going to remind you anyway, since it's a rant I make regularly to my daughters! Greens tend to be low in calories but high in so many vitamins and minerals, especially calcium, which of course promotes bone health and is particularly important in dairy-free diets. Go exotic with superfoods in our Broccoli and Coconut with Red Lentils, get your protein hit with our Hearty Pea and Lentil, or go for an immune boost with our Courgette and Watercress Pesto. You can really take your health to the next level by going green.

This is the sort of soup where you gather up what's hanging around in your fridge on a summer's day and turn those slightly curled-up vegetables and leaves into something stunning. You'll create a soup that's light and refreshing, perfect for helping you shape up for summer and full of the delights of a British country garden. What's more, if you can grow some of the produce yourself, you'll also have the pleasure of knowing the provenance of what you're eating. This soup is light on calories, high on fibre and big on taste!

ENGLISH SUMMER VEGETABLES

Serves 4

2 tbsp rapeseed oil

100 g (3½ oz) frozen peas

2½ spring onions, trimmed and chopped

2 medium potatoes, peeled and chopped

500 ml (16 fl oz) vegetable stock

½ iceberg lettuce, trimmed and diced

¼ cucumber, washed and sliced

1 fresh mint leaf

Salt and freshly ground black pepper

Pea shoots (optional)

Heat the oil in a pan and add the peas, spring onion and potato. Cook gently for 3–4 minutes.

Add the vegetable stock to the vegetables and bring to the boil. Lower the heat and simmer, partially covered, until the potato pieces are tender; this will take around 20 minutes.

Take off the heat and blend until completely smooth.

Add the lettuce, cucumber and mint, return to the heat and simmer for a further 2 minutes.

Remove from the heat, blend until completely smooth, season to taste and serve. Decorate with a sprig of mint or a pea shoot or two.

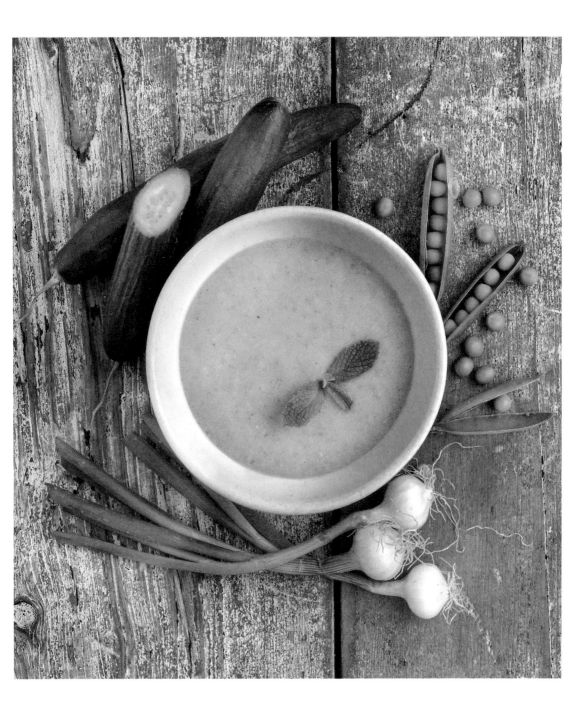

A combination of broccoli and red lentils might seem surprising, but this recipe really works! The blend of the green and the red results in an interesting colour but this soup is fantastic body fuel and super-tasty as well. It's important to blend the soup well in order to create its distinctive thick, creamy texture, which comes from the lentils. As we note elsewhere, broccoli is an undercover superfood, which contains high levels of betacarotene, vitamins C, D, and K, and calcium too – all of which promote good bone health. It is a powerful detoxer too, having three glucosinolate phytonutrients that help neutralise and eliminate contaminants in the body. And if that weren't enough, broccoli and lentils are both fibre-rich, which is important for maintaining good digestive health.

BROCCOLI AND COCONUT WITH RED LENTILS

Serves 4–5

2 tbsp rapeseed oil

1 medium onion, chopped

3 garlic cloves, peeled and chopped

¼ tsp mild chilli powder

550 g (1¼ lb) broccoli (heads and stems), trimmed and chopped

140 g (5 oz) dried red lentils

1 litre (1¾ pints) vegetable stock

125 g (4½ oz) coconut cream

Salt and freshly ground black pepper

Caramelise the onion in the oil (see page 34), then add the garlic, chilli powder and broccoli and let the vegetables sweat for 5–6 minutes, partially covered. Stir occasionally.

Wash and drain the lentils, then add them to the vegetables and mix in well. Add the vegetable stock, stir well and bring to the boil.

Turn down the heat and simmer gently, until the lentils are completely cooked, stirring regularly to make sure the lentils do not stick to the bottom of the pan.

Add the coconut cream and mix in well. Take off the heat and blend the soup until completely smooth. Season to taste.

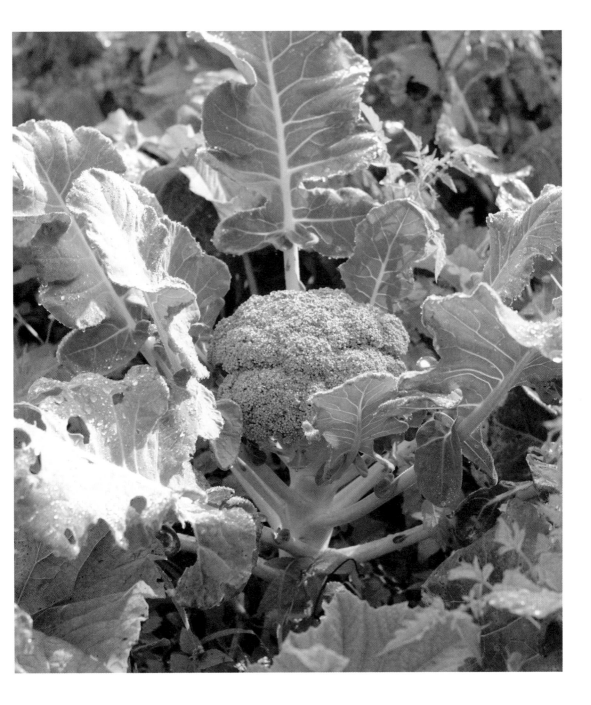

Superfoods are springing up all around these days, with every vegetable, fruit, nut and grain wanting to get in on the act. This is no surprise, really, when you consider that being classified as a superfood can send sales rocketing into the stratosphere. However, not all superfoods are created equal and sometimes the simplest ones are the best. Broccoli, please take centre stage – no more hanging around forlornly at the edge of the plate for you! With so much going for it, what with its anti-inflammatory properties, high vitamin count and new research suggesting it can help lower the risk of stroke and heart disease, broccoli truly deserves its superfood accolade. Here, a little bit of almond pesto drizzled over the soup gives this hero vegetable some well-deserved pizzazz.

BROCCOLI SOUP WITH ALMOND PESTO

Serves 4–6

For the soup

2 tbsp rapeseed oil

550 g (1¼ lb) broccoli (heads and stems), washed and finely chopped

1 litre (1¾ pints) vegetable stock

Salt and freshly ground black pepper

For the pesto

5 tbsp olive oil

1 garlic clove, peeled and finely chopped

1 tbsp chopped broccoli florets

15 g (½ oz) ground almonds

Pinch of salt

Chop sufficient tips from the broccoli florets to use for the pesto and set aside.

Prepare the soup: gently sauté the remaining broccoli in the rapeseed oil for around 5 minutes, until the broccoli becomes tender. Add the vegetable stock and bring to the boil.

Turn down the heat and simmer, partially covered, for around 8 minutes, until the broccoli is soft but not overcooked. Stir frequently. Take off the heat and blend until completely smooth. Season to taste.

To make the almond pesto: put all the ingredients together into a bowl, mix together, then blend until smooth.

To serve, put the broccoli soup into some pretty bowls and drizzle a generous swirl of the almond pesto on the top.

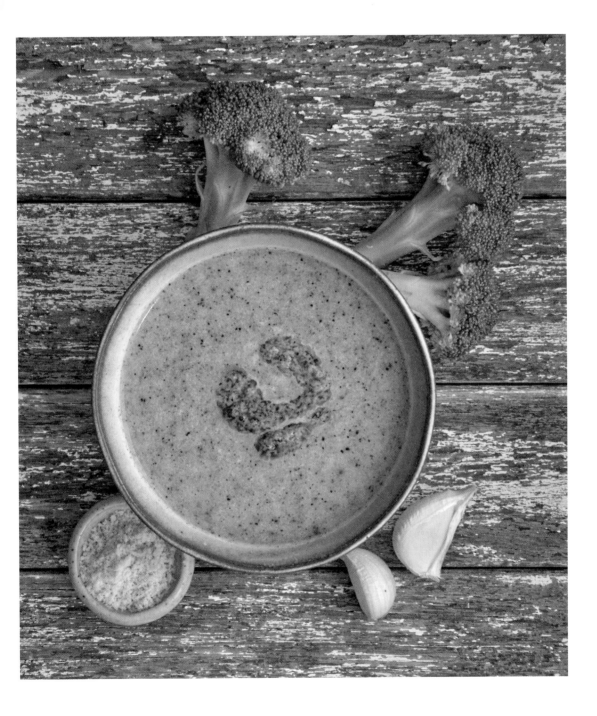

Cabbage still gets a bad rap and I'm convinced it's because it is so often served up overcooked and therefore tasteless. I'm hoping this soup will help you obliterate bad memories and convert you to enjoying this unassuming veggie! Unlike the infamous cabbage soup of old, which contained nothing but those dense leaves cooked into a foul-smelling broth, this soup contains a delicious savoury mix. The kale provides a wonderful depth of flavour, while the caraway seeds give the soup a pleasant, fragrant undertone. The carrots, garlic and leeks add a natural sweetness to the whole dish. All these ingredients help to make the cabbage itself shine, so it becomes a treat rather than torture. It may also help to know that cabbage is full of nutrients, including vitamins C, K and B6, as well as being a great source of folate. Top with some sprouting alfalfa for extra texture, if you like.

CABBAGE AND KALE SOUP

Serves 5–6

2 tbsp rapeseed oil

1 large onion, chopped

2 small leeks, chopped

3 garlic cloves, peeled and chopped

2 large carrots, peeled and chopped

1 medium potato, peeled and chopped

200 g (7 oz) Savoy cabbage, finely shredded

65 g (2¼ oz) kale

1 tsp caraway seeds

1.5 litres (2¾ pints) vegetable stock

Salt and freshly ground black pepper

Caramelise the onion in the oil (see *page 34*), then add the leeks and garlic.

Cook, partially covered, for 2–3 minutes, then add the carrots, potato, cabbage, kale and caraway seeds.

Let the vegetables sweat for 5–6 minutes, partially covered. Stir occasionally.

Add the vegetable stock and bring to the boil. Then turn down the heat and simmer gently, partially covered, for around 8–10 minutes, until the carrots and potato are soft. Give the soup an occasional stir.

When cooked, take off the heat and blend the soup until completely smooth. Season to taste.

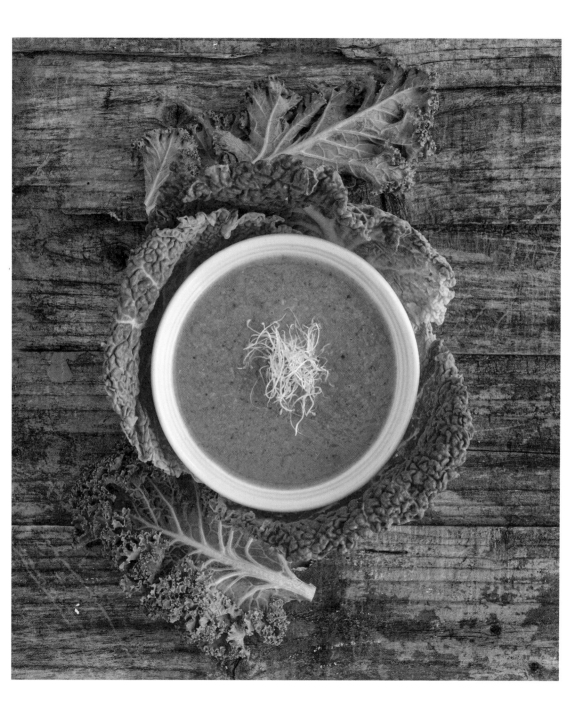

I love this soup, because it's a bit of a show-stopper; the vibrant green courgette base has a dash of dark green pesto poised on the top for maximum effect. Tastewise, when you mix the two together, it's a sensational hit! The natural pepperiness of the watercress gives a real kick, which is needed, I think, as courgettes on their own can be a little bland. Try to buy small rather than large courgettes – you'll end up with a sweeter and more succulent dish. This soup is perfect for any healthy eating regime, with the raw watercress pesto providing a wonderful hit of iron.

COURGETTE WITH WATERCRESS PESTO

Serves 3–4

For the soup

2 tbsp rapeseed oil

1 onion, chopped

1 garlic clove, peeled and chopped

1 small potato, peeled and chopped

450 g (1 lb) courgettes, trimmed and sliced (but unpeeled)

850 ml (1½ pints) vegetable stock

Salt and freshly ground black pepper

For the pesto

50 g (1¾ oz) watercress (including stalks)

1 garlic clove, peeled and chopped

3 tsp sunflower seeds

2 tsp sesame seeds

½ tsp salt

180 ml (6 fl oz) olive oill

Caramelise the onion in the oil (*see page 34*), then add the garlic, potato and courgette. Let the vegetables sweat for 5–6 minutes, partially covered, stirring occasionally.

Add the vegetable stock and bring to the boil. Then turn down the heat and simmer gently, partially covered, for around 10 minutes, until the potato pieces are soft. Stir occasionally.

While the vegetables are cooking, put all the ingredients for the pesto into a container together and blend until completely emulsified, then set aside.

Once the soup is ready, take off the heat and blend the soup until completely smooth. Season to taste.

Serve by pouring the soup into a bowl and swirling some of the pesto into the centre.

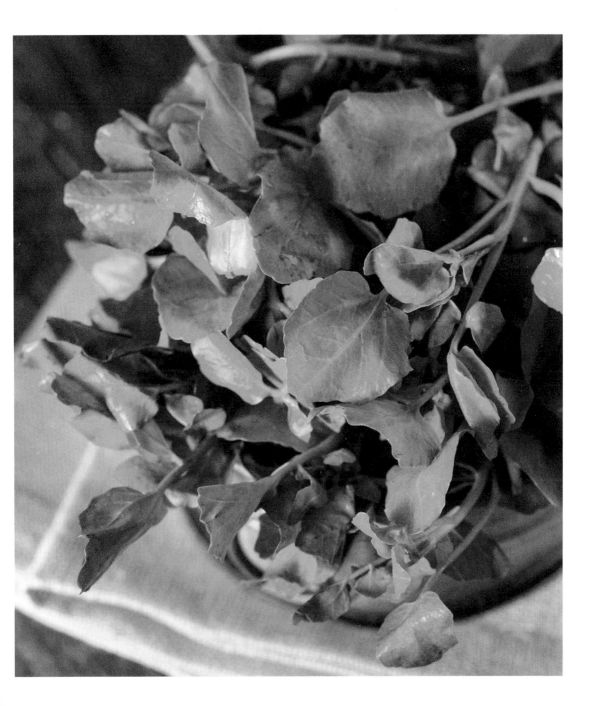

KALE AND APPLE SOUP WITH WALNUT AND CIDER PESTO

Serves 4–5

For the pesto

45 g (1½ oz) pumpkin seeds

1½ tbsp rapeseed oil

4 walnuts, halved

70 ml (1¾ fl oz) medium-dry cider

Salt and freshly ground black pepper

For the soup

2 tbsp rapeseed oil

1 large onion, chopped

1 garlic clove, peeled and chopped

2 carrots, peeled and chopped

2 eating apples, cored and chopped (unpeeled)

1.25 litres (2 pints) vegetable stock

200 g (7 oz) kale, roughly chopped

Salt and freshly ground black pepper

Begin by toasting the pumpkin seeds for the pesto. Pre-heat the oven to 150°C/300°F/Gas Mark 2. Line a small baking tray with baking parchment and add the pumpkin seeds. Sprinkle a small amount of oil over the seeds, then mix well and spread the seeds evenly on the tray. Bake in the oven for about 40 minutes, until the seeds are turning a golden brown.

While the seeds are cooking, caramelise the onion in the oil (see page 34). Then add the garlic and the carrots and continue to cook on a low heat for 4–5 minutes, partially covered.

Add the apples and cook for a further 2–3 minutes, partially covered. Add the stock, stir well and bring to the boil.

Turn down the heat, add the kale and simmer gently, partially covered, for around 7 minutes, until the carrots are cooked. Stir occasionally.

Begin blending with the heat still on, for 3–4 minutes, then allow the soup to simmer for another 3–4 minutes. Take off the heat and blend the soup again, until completely smooth. Season to taste.

To make the pesto, put the toasted pumpkin seeds, walnuts and cider into a bowl or beaker and blend until smooth. If too thick, add a little more oil and blend again. Season to taste.

To serve, spoon a couple of generous tablespoons of the pesto over each bowl of soup.

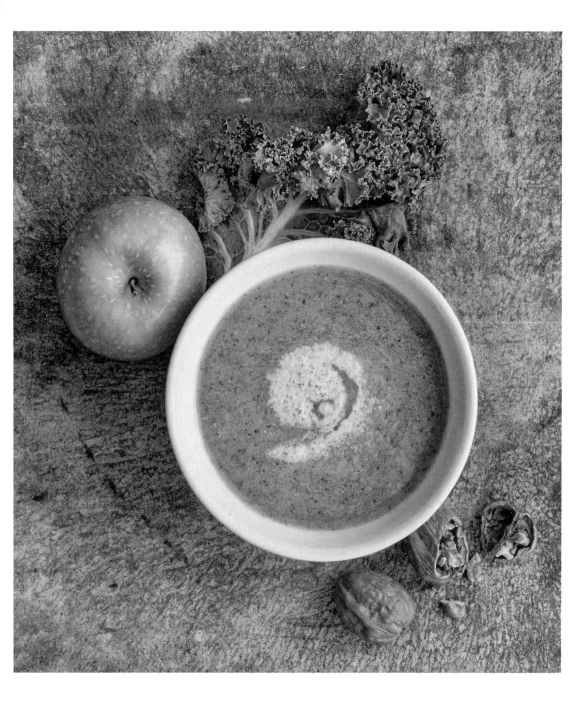

Leeks are a member of the allium family, along with onions and garlic, so they have the same wonderful combination of flavonoids and sulphur-containing nutrients. Just one cup of cooked leeks will provide you with 29 per cent of your Vitamin K daily requirement. Leeks are sweet too, taking the slight bitterness off the mushrooms. If you leave the mushrooms in the sunshine for half an hour before using them, you'll benefit from the added Vitamin D they'll soak up too.

LEEK AND MUSHROOM

Serves 4

2 tbsp rapeseed oil

I small onion, chopped

I clove of garlic, chopped

2 leeks, finely sliced

50 g (1¾ oz) fresh Portobello or Portobellini mushrooms

100 g (3½ oz) button or cup mushrooms

¼ tsp dried thyme

750 ml (1¼ pints) vegetable stock

I tbsp fresh lime juice

Salt and freshly ground black pepper

Caramelise the onion in the oil (see *page 34*).

Add the garlic and leeks, and sauté them lightly with the onion before adding the mushrooms and thyme. Cook on a medium to low heat until the vegetables become tender, stirring occasionally.

Pour in the vegetable stock and bring to the boil, then lower the heat and allow to simmer, partially covered, for 8 minutes, or until the vegetables are completely soft.

Add the lime juice, mix it in well and take the pan off the heat.

Blend the soup until completely smooth and season to taste.

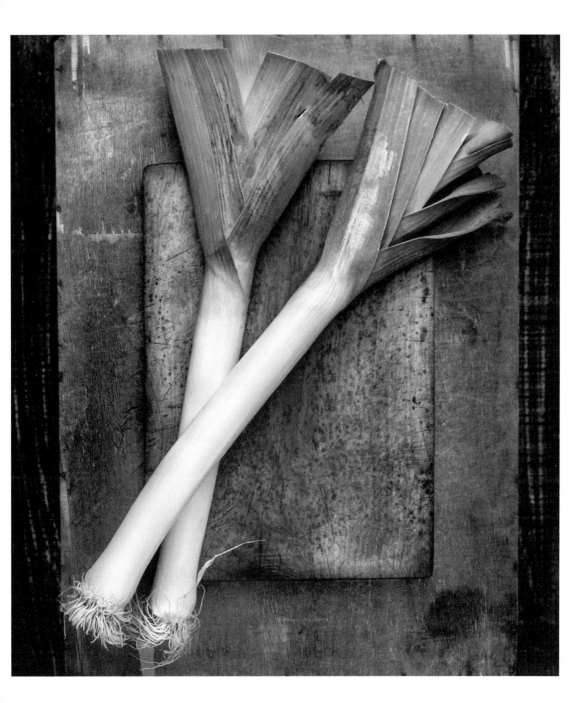

This is the soup I always wheel out when the girls are back from uni and we're pretty sure they haven't eaten properly for at least a month. Hearty by name, hearty by nature, this thick creamy soup will fill you up with protein, fibre and general goodness. It leaves you feeling happy and satisfied and – even though I'm pretty sure nothing can do this – I like to pretend that this soup makes up for all the late nights and lack of decent nutrition the girls have undergone in the previous weeks. As I don't dilute the soup by adding any milk or cream, every mouthful is packed with nourishment, so it really is a great soup to help build back strength and stamina if you've had a few extra stresses and strains.

HEARTY PEA AND LENTIL

Serves 4–6

2 tbsp rapeseed oil

I small onion, chopped

I clove of garlic, chopped

I small leek, sliced finely

3 celery sticks, trimmed and chopped

125 g (4½ oz) frozen peas

250 g (9 oz) dried red split lentils

1.25 litres (2 pints) vegetable stock

I tsp fresh lime juice

Salt and freshly ground black pepper

Caramelise the onion in the oil (see *page 34*).

Add the garlic, leeks and celery, and place over a medium to low heat, partially covered. Cook until the vegetables become tender, stirring occasionally.

Wash and drain the lentils. Add the peas and lentils to the vegetables, and stir in well before pouring in the vegetable stock and bringing to the boil.

Turn down the heat and simmer gently, partially covered, for around 20 minutes, or until the lentils are completely cooked. Stir occasionally.

Mix in the lime juice and then blend the soup until completely smooth. Take off the heat, season to taste and serve.

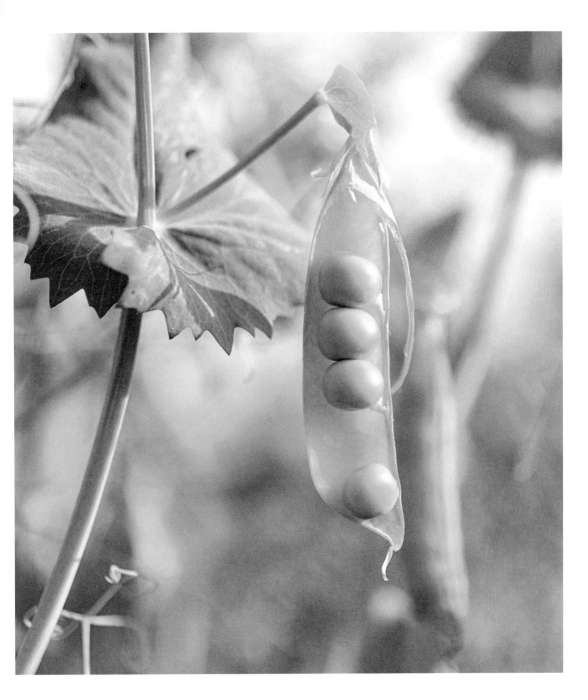

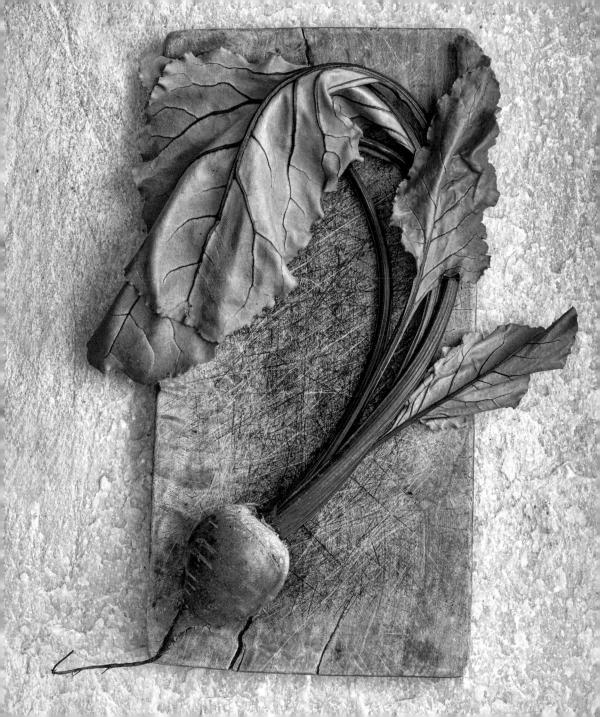

THE PURPLE SOUPS

My purple collection of soups makes for a
strikingly pretty display that tastes just as good as
it looks. My personal hero is beetroot, dazzling in
both colour and health benefits, with its vitamins,
anti-inflammatories and antioxidants. Pick your
purple veg carefully – size really does matter, and
bigger isn't always better, with smaller vegetables
often being sweeter and more succulent. Try your
hand at beetroot with my Beetroot and Rhubarb
soup or the Purple Soup. If you're feeling in need
of a sweetener, why not go for a little Blueberry?

There's no other name for this soup! It looks divine and tastes fabulous too. The red cabbage and beetroot provide the robust, earthy flavour, which is contrasted with the sweetness of the dried cranberry. On a nutritional note, this soup is filled with wonders: red cabbage contains high levels of betacarotene, which is essential for eye and bone health, and a powerful antioxidant; beetroot is known for its blood-pressure-lowering benefits (when combined with a healthy lifestyle) as well as containing a wide array of minerals and vitamins, such as calcium and iron; and, finally, cranberries are high in Vitamin C. This is high-powered fuel in the form of purple delicousness. Dot with chia seeds on serving for fun, fibre and lots of extra minerals.

PURPLE SOUP

Serves 3–4

2 tbsp rapeseed oil

1 large onion, chopped

1 medium beetroot, peeled and chopped

100 g (3½ oz) red cabbage, chopped

1 litre (1¾ pints) vegetable stock

50 g (1¾ oz) dried cranberries

Salt and freshly ground black pepper

Caramelise the onion in the oil (see page 34), then add the beetroot and red cabbage and let the vegetables sweat for 5–6 minutes, partially covered. Stir occasionally.

Add the vegetable stock, stir well and bring to the boil.

Turn down the heat, add the dried cranberries, partially cover and allow to simmer gently for around 20 minutes, until the beetroot is soft. Stir occasionally. .

Take off the heat and blend the soup until completely smooth. Season to taste.

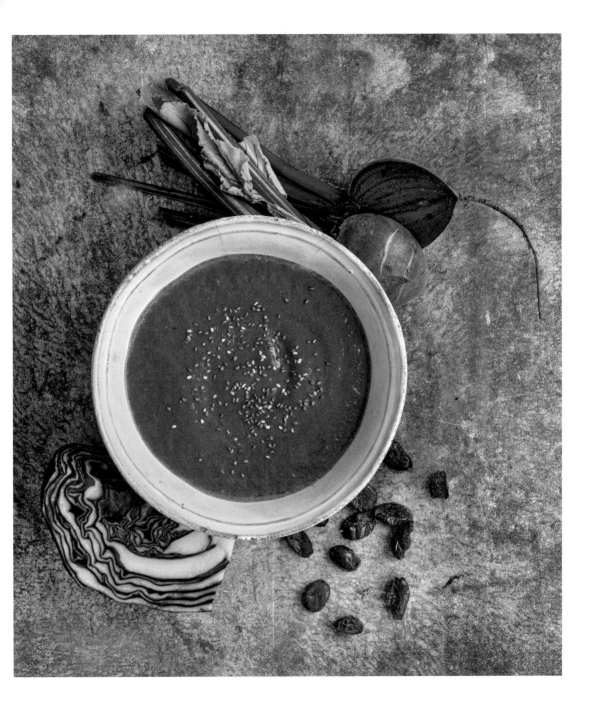

A lot of people say that they don't like beetroot, but I think that the natural blend of sweetness and earthiness is delicious when balanced carefully with the other ingredients that I've included in this recipe. Several studies have confirmed that the betalains (nitrogen-containing pigments) and nitrates in beetroots are exceptionally good for you, particularly in helping to lower blood pressure. Don't be concerned if the colour of the soup changes; the beetroot colour, which makes it high in betacarotene, is volatile and can be affected by temperature, both hot and cold. The colour can also vary according to the variety of beetroot you're using.

BEETROOT AND ORANGE

Serves 4

5 beetroots, peeled and roughly chopped

3 garlic cloves, whole and unpeeled

8 sprigs fresh thyme

3 strips orange zest

4 tbsp rapeseed oil

750 ml (1¼ pints) vegetable stock

75 ml (2½ fl oz) fresh orange juice

2 tsp agave nectar

Salt and freshly ground black pepper

Preheat the oven to 190°C/375°F/Gas mark 5.

Line a roasting tin with aluminium foil and arrange the beetroot, garlic, thyme and orange zest on top. Sprinkle over the oil and mix well, then tightly cover with foil. Roast in the oven for 20–25 minutes.

Remove from the oven, allow to cool for a few minutes, then remove the thyme, discard the orange zest, and carefully squeeze out the contents of the garlic cloves. Discard the skins.

Transfer the contents of the roasting tin into a saucepan and place on a medium to low heat. Add the vegetable stock, mix in well, then partially cover and bring to the boil. Then lower the heat and let it simmer, partially covered, for around 10 minutes, until the beetroot is soft.

Add the orange juice and agave nectar, stir well, then take off the heat. Blend until completely smooth. Season to taste.

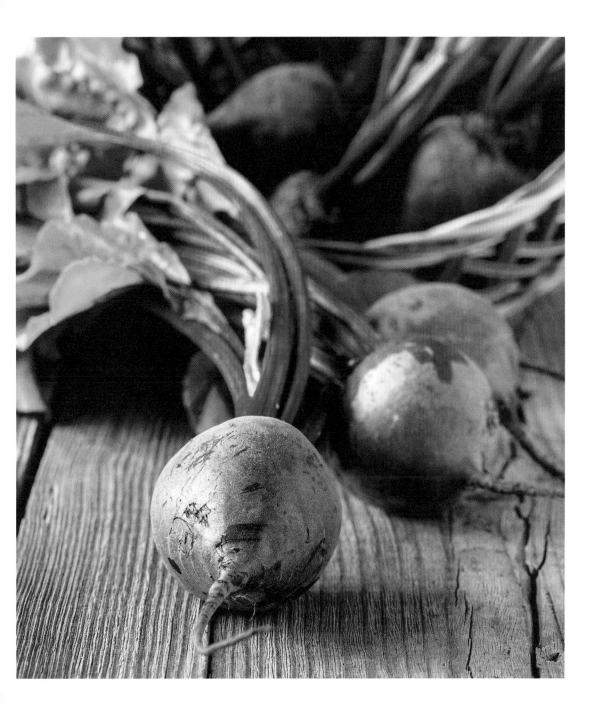

The rich flavours of beetroot and rhubarb are tied together here by the addition of orange, which is a fruit that beautifully crosses the sweet-to-savoury boundary. The orange in this soup provides the Vitamin C hit, while the beetroot contains nitrates that can help to lower blood pressure when combined with a healthy lifestyle. The rhubarb is a good source of vitamins A and K. This soup is delicious chilled or hot, topped with some parsnip crisps (*see page 52*).

BEETROOT AND RHUBARB

Serves 5–6

For the rhubarb purée
450 g (1 lb) rhubarb stalks
60 ml (2 fl oz) fresh orange juice

For the soup
2 tbsp rapeseed oil
1 large onion, chopped
3 medium beetroots, peeled and chopped
250 g (9 oz) swede, peeled and chopped
1 large carrot, peeled and chopped
1 medium parsnip, peeled and chopped
250 g (9 oz) red cabbage, chopped
1.25 litres (2 pints) vegetable stock
¼ teaspoon mustard powder
2 tsp grated orange zest
Salt and freshly ground black pepper

Put the rhubarb in a pan with the orange juice and cook for 5–6 minutes on a medium heat, until soft. Set aside and allow to cool.

In a separate pan, caramelise the onion in the oil (*see page 34*).

Add the beetroot, swede, carrot, parsnip and red cabbage, and let the vegetables sweat for 5–6 minutes, partially covered over a low to medium heat. Stir occasionally.

Add the vegetable stock and mustard, and stir well. Bring to the boil, then turn down the heat and simmer gently, partially covered, for around 20 minutes, until the vegetables are soft. Stir from time to time during cooking.

Add the cooked rhubarb, including any juice, and the orange zest and mix well. Take off the heat and blend the soup until completely smooth. Season to taste.

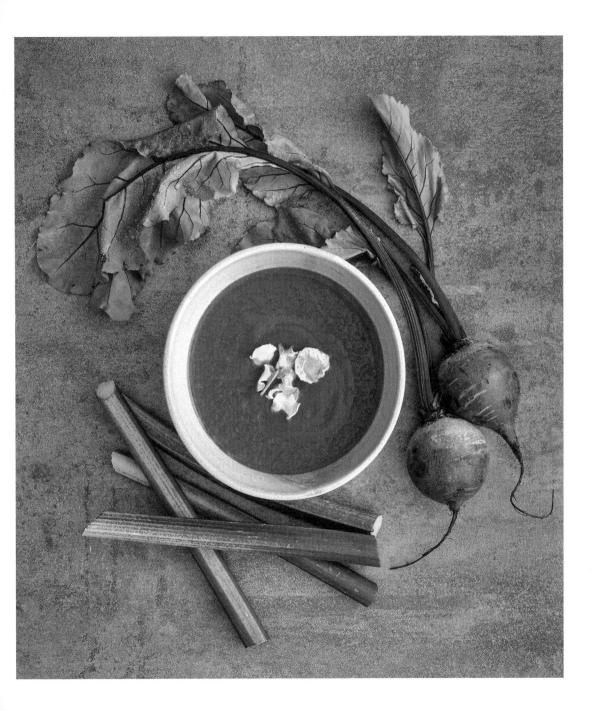

Here I have turned the iconic superfood into a delicious 'souper' food. Sweet yet tangy, this soup is a hit even with those who won't usually go near the nutrient-packed blueberry. A little cooking tip is called for here, which is well worth following, unless you want to play a game of 'clove or blueberry husk?' with the finished soup. Before adding the lemons and cloves to the pan, stud the cloves into the lemon slices. This makes it much easier to locate the cloves amongst the dark colour of the blueberry soup when you're ready to remove them.

BLUEBERRY SOUP

Serves 4

2 slices lemon

2 cloves, whole

400 g (14 oz) blueberries

5 cm (2 in) cinnamon stick

1.5 tbsp fresh lemon juice

1 tbsp cornflour

Maple syrup or agave nectar (optional)

Stud the lemon skin with the cloves and place with the blueberries, cinnamon stick, and 750 ml (1¼ pints) water in a pan. Bring to the boil, then turn down the heat and simmer for 10–15 minutes until the blueberries are soft.

Remove the lemon slices, cloves and cinnamon stick and discard. Put the remaining mixture into a blender and process until smooth.

Pour the blended mixture back into the pan and add the lemon juice.

In a cup, mix the cornflour with a little cold water to create a smooth paste. Slowly add to the soup, gradually bringing it to the boil, stirring constantly until the soup has thickened. When you initially add the cornflour, it will make the soup go opaque, but as it cooks though (coming to the boil then back to a simmer), the soup will become clear again, having thickened at the same time. Add your chosen sweetener to taste.

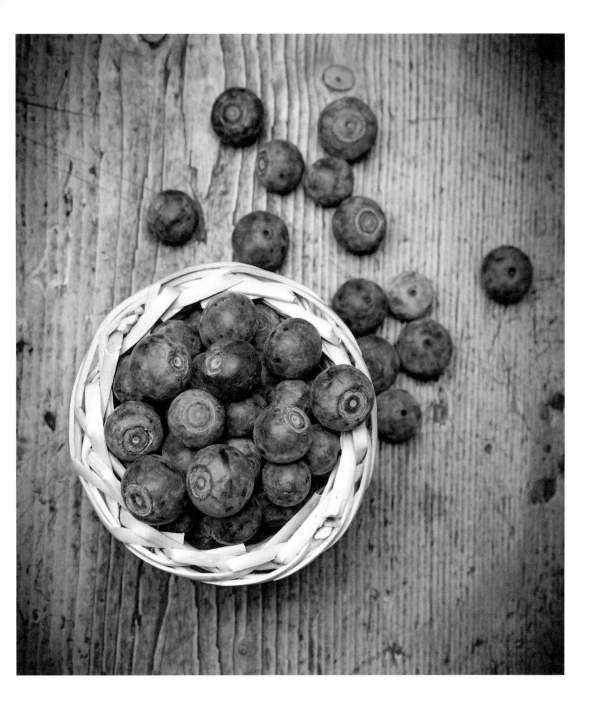

INDEX

ACKNOWLEDGEMENTS

AUTHOR CREDITS

This book would never have seen the light of day without the love and support of my wife, Amanda; daughters, Fredericka, Victoria, Henrietta and Anastasia, son-in-law, Jeremy, and all their friends who make up our unofficial taste testers. Huge thanks to Giulia Sciota, Grace Magecha and Vanessa Roster for their incredible help and patience. I would also like to thank Philly Vass for her tremendous assistance; Sian Porter, consultant dietitian and Katherine Kimber, for all their advice, along with Hannah Meur, for her amazing designs, past and future. I am very grateful to my agent, Amanda Preston, as well as Katy Denny and the wonderful team at Vermillion for their help, support and encouragement. Thanks also go to Sarah Tomley and Tracy Killick for their brilliant creative skills. Finally, I would like to thank Soupologistas everywhere who support & believe.

PUBLISHER CREDIT

The Publishers would like to thank the wonderful creative team at North Street Potters, London, for the loan of their beautiful handmade bowls. www.northstreetpotters.com

PICTURE CREDITS

Every effort has been made to contact copyright holders. However, the publishers will be glad to rectify in future editions any inadvertent omissions brought to their attention.

123RF Vicushka 15; Akulamatiau 37; Noam Armonn 79; Natalia Zakharova 103; Arthit Buarapa 132; Victoria Shibut 143; Oksana Tkachuk 145; Vera Kuttelvaserova Stuchelova 155.

Dreamstime Lunamarina 19; Diego Vito Cervo 34; Catherine O'Keefe 56; Steven Cukrov 66; Loonara 71; Ian Andreiev 85; Christian Jung 105; Bhofack2 139; Istetiana 151.

iStockphoto Tanjamy 12; Ihar Ulashchyk 16tr; Knape 16br; Ehaurylik 21; Sturti 23; JohnnyMad 32; DebbiSmirnoff 32; Scottshotz 36; Lena Sergeeva 59; Jatrax 68; RapidEye 83; Alison Stieglitz 89; Anna1311 92; Letty17 99; Eli Asenova 103; Bojsha65 117; Leekris 127.

Shutterstock Igorsm8 40; Kunanon 49; Artpritsadee 75.

Soupologie 7tl, tr, br, bl, m; 11; 16l.

Thinkstock Bart Kowski 29; Merc67 35; GJohnstonphoto 47.

Commissioning Editor **Katy Denny**

Managing Editor **Sarah Tomley**

Art Director **Tracy Killick**

Production Manager **Lucy Harrison**

Photographer **Jean Cazals**

Food stylist **Marie-Ange Lapierre**

Illustrator **Hannah Meur**

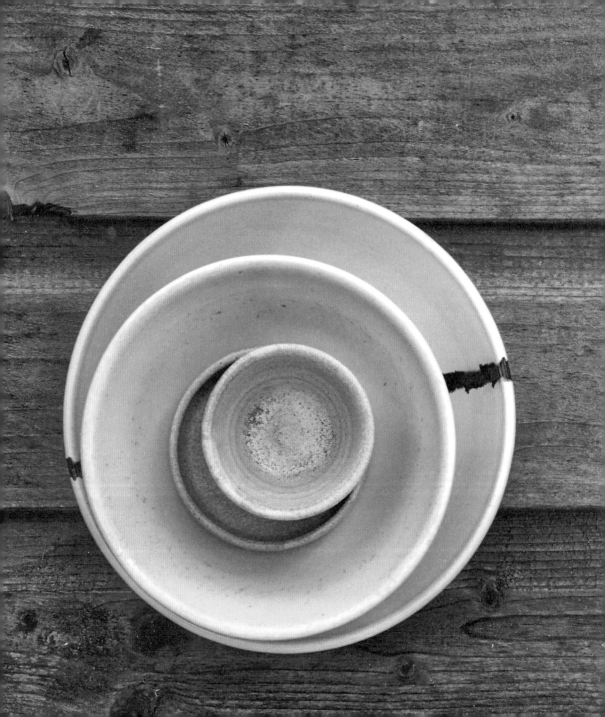